RENAL AND UROLOGIC DISORDERS

PERITONEAL DIALYSIS

TYPES, PROCEDURES AND RISKS FACTORS

RENAL AND UROLOGIC DISORDERS

Additional books in this series can be found on Nova's website under the Series tab.

Additional e-books in this series can be found on Nova's website under the e-book tab.

PUBLIC HEALTH IN THE 21ST CENTURY

Additional books in this series can be found on Nova's website under the Series tab.

Additional e-books in this series can be found on Nova's website under the e-book tab.

RENAL AND UROLOGIC DISORDERS

PERITONEAL DIALYSIS

TYPES, PROCEDURES AND RISKS FACTORS

ANIL K. AGARWAL
LOAY SALMAN
AND
ARIF ASIF
EDITORS

NOVA BIOMEDICAL
New York

For permission to use material from this book please contact us:
Telephone 631-231-7269; Fax 631-231-8175
Web Site: http://www.novapublishers.com

Library of Congress Cataloging-in-Publication Data

ISBN: 978-1-62257-896-2

Library of Congress Control Number: 2012947892

Published by Nova Science Publishers, Inc. † New York

CONTENTS

INTRODUCTION

The book 'Peritoneal Dialysis: Types, Procedures and Risks Factors' presents a compilation of concise and pertinent discussion of hot topics related to this important, but often ignored, modality of dialysis. The chapters review important literature to provide insight into the mechanisms and technical aspects of peritoneal dialysis (PD). PD is a harshly underutilized modality of renal replacement. Continuous PD can enjoy weekly solute clearances approaching those with hemodialysis. Recent clinical research data indicates at least an initial survival advantage as well as better preservation of residual renal function of patients started on PD as compared to those initiated on hemodialysis. Recent advances in knowledge of mechanisms and new technological advances including development of advanced dialysis solutions have potential to improvise PD to extend its initial survival advantage to long-term treatment.

Peritoneal membrane is the lifeline for PD patients. Permeability or transport status of the membrane is usually measured by doing a Peritoneal Equilibration Test. Peritoneal transport status at the commencement of PD predicts risks of technique failure and death and can facilitate better assessment, diagnosis and therapeutic management of PD complications. As we better understand the mechanisms of injury and functional responses, therapies to improve clinical outcomes may evolve.

PD related infections are a major cause of morbidity and mortality in patients with end-stage kidney disease. Prevention, early recognition and adequate management of these infections are of paramount importance. Exit site, tunnel infections and CAPD-associated peritonitis need to be differentiated and aggressively treated. Despite technology advances, prevention of peritonitis remains one of the major challenges in PD. Several innovative developments have shown an impact on peritonitis rates including antimicrobial-coated catheter modifications and topical application of antimicrobial agents. New alternative agents for topical exit-site care with reduced potential for antimicrobial resistance are under development. Flushing before fill and avoidance of spiking of solution bags has improved peritonitis rates, as have innovative connectology and double-bag systems. The incidence of peritonitis has markedly improved since the end of the 1980s, but infection remains a significant complication of chronic PD.

PD offers capability to optimize extracellular fluid management in the context of abnormal autoregulation, commonly encountered in patients with congestive heart failure (CHF). Slow, continuous ultrafiltration, has been utilized in CHF in patients with and without other indications for kidney replacement therapy. PD can serve as a viable choice for these patients.

Finally, high glucose concentration of PD fluid can be associated with non-infectious complications of PD, including worsening of glycemia, apart from causing damage to the peritoneal membrane, altering its physiologic characteristics, often leading to the failure of this technique. Control of hyperglycemia can be achieved via diet and weight restrictions, use of non-glucose PD solutions such as icodextrin and use of fewer daily exchanges of low-glucose solutions.

In: Peritoneal Dialysis
Editors: A. Agarwal, L. Salman et al.
ISBN: 978-1-62257-896-2

Chapter 1

Peritoneal Dialysis: An Overview

I-Wen Wu[1,2], Chi-Jen Tsai[1,2,3], Shyh-Chuan Jwo[2,4,5] and Mai-Szu Wu[1,2*]

[1] Department of Nephrology, Chang Gung Memorial Hospital, Keelung, Taiwan
[2] School of Medicine, Chang Gung University
[3] School of Medicine, Taipei Medical University
[4] Division of General Surgery, Chang Gung Memorial Hospital, Keelung, Taiwan
[5] Institute of Bioscience and Biotechnology, National Taiwan Ocean University, Keelung, Taiwan

Abstract

Several different techniques are available for performing peritoneal dialysis (PD). The rates of peritoneal blood flow and dialysate flow with PD are well below those achieved with hemodialysis (where both are often above 400 mL/min). Thus, the clearance of urea and other small solutes per unit time is much less with PD than with hemodialysis. However, PD is often performed in a continuous fashion so that the weekly solute clearances approach those with hemodialysis.

* E-mail address: yamamasa1155@yahoo.co.jp

TYPES OF PD

PD can be performed in a continuous or intermittent fashion [1].

Continuous ambulatory peritoneal dialysis (CAPD) involves multiple exchanges during the day (usually three) followed by an overnight dwell. A modification involves one nighttime exchange with an exchange device, resulting in two overnight exchanges and three exchanges during the day [2]. CAPD can be used, with a typical minimum dialysis prescription of four, two liter exchanges per day, including one overnight exchange. This standard regimen can be modified by changing either dwell time, volume or the number of exchanges per day. The exchanges are performed manually.

Automated peritoneal dialysis (APD) usually consists of continuous cycler peritoneal dialysis (CCPD), nightly intermittent peritoneal dialysis (NIPD), and tidal peritoneal dialysis (TPD) [3]. In comparison, APD is an automated form of therapy in which a cycler delivers 3 to 6 exchanges while the patient sleeps with a 12 to 15 hour daytime dwell. Weekly clearances are similar to those obtained with CAPD but more dialysate fluid is generally required each day.

- **Continuous cycler peritoneal dialysis (CCPD)** has a long daytime dwell and several cycles overnight. A minority of those undergoing CCPD do not have a daytime dwell and some patients must do a daytime or midday exchange [2].
- **Nightly intermittent peritoneal dialysis (NIPD) or intermittent peritoneal dialysis (IPD)** are intermittent techniques with some treatment periods ("wet" abdomen) alternating with times during which the peritoneal cavity has been drained of dialysate ("dry" abdomen). Classic IPD is a form of dialysis in which multiple short exchanges are performed on an intermittent basis. A typical regimen consists of 12 to 15 two liter, one hour dwells performed three or four days per week. Over 50 hours of dialysis are required to attain clearances similar to CAPD. However, even higher target doses of dialysis are recommended because of the peaks in BUN occurring on the off-dialysis days. For these reasons, this form of PD is not recommended for chronic use.

- **Tidal peritoneal dialysis (TPD)**, consists of exchanges in which the peritoneal cavity always contains at least some dialysate (usually one-half full), a feature that improves comfort and facilitates drainage in some patients [4]. The patient may or may not have a daytime dwell.

The intermittent regimens typically utilize multiple short dwells and automated technology to operate at near maximum solute clearance rates. Of the intermittent techniques, TPD is infrequently used because it is very expensive (requires a large number of dialysate) and is technically difficult to perform. Increased solute clearances have also not been confirmed in patients, despite such findings in animal models [2,5]. Most frequently, TPD is used to minimize drainage problems in selected patients. As recommended in the European Best Practice guidelines, it can also be used in those with inflow/outflow pain and in patients with slow peritoneal drainage [6].

Continuous flow peritoneal dialysis (CFPD) is another technique in which two peritoneal catheters or one catheter with two ports provide the continuous inflow and outflow of dialysate [7]. Since the dialysate is constantly refreshed, clearances similar to that obtained with daily hemodialysis can be obtained. CFPD was first introduced decades ago, but was subsequently abandoned because of technical and financial limitations. However, in a crossover study of five patients found that CFPD enhanced diffusive transport and the mean ultrafiltration rate compared with nightly intermittent PD and nightly tidal PD [8]. Additional study is required to better understand the practicality of this technique.

At the start of dialysis when patients have some residual renal function, most patients could do any PD technique and usually be able to achieve the Kt/V and volume control targets. However, once residual kidney function is negligible, modality choice may need to match peritoneal transport characteristics to optimize solute clearance and ultrafiltration. It is important to individualize the patient's dwell times and dwell volumes so that the target dose of PD can be achieved. As an example, PD is considered adequate in most patients if the weekly total Kt/V for urea is at least 1.7 and, if considering creatinine clearance, the weekly creatinine clearance is at least 50 to 60 L/week per 1.73 m2 body surface area (with some variation based upon transporter status). Attainment of these goals must be documented and then monitored over time. It is often necessary, for example, to increase the patient's dialysis prescription (usually by increasing the number of exchanges or the dwell volume) as residual renal function is lost or there is a decrease in the net permeability of the peritoneal membrane. However, in spite of paucity of data, CAPD and APD appear to provide similar clinical outcomes [9-12]. A systematic review of three randomized controlled trials including 139 patients undergoing either APD or CAPD found that both PD modalities resulted in similar mortality and hospitalization rates, risk of peritonitis, fluid leaks, and effect upon residual renal function. APD may be associated with relatively more time for work and social activities [9,10]. Another prospective multicenter cohort five-year study of 87 APD and 562 CAPD patients showed that overall mortality and the incidence of technique failure were the same with both techniques [11]. Several factors are important determinants of PD modality choice.

Peritoneal equilibration test

The first step in optimizing a PD prescription is to determine the peritoneal membrane transport characteristics using the peritoneal equilibration test [13]. Based upon published norms, the patient's transport characteristics are classified into “rapid” or “slow”transporters. The dwell time is then matched to the transport type in an effort to maximize daily clearances and ultrafiltration while minimizing glucose absorption [14]. The patients with rapid transporters achieve almost total equilibration between plasma and dialysate for urea and creatinine in a few hours. They also are rapid absorbers of dialysate glucose, thereby removing the osmotic stimulus to ultrafiltration. The net effect is that they begin to absorb dialysate with the glucose leading, after two to three hours, to reductions in ultrafiltration volume and net solute clearance (as the solutes that have diffused into the dialysate are also absorbed back into the systemic circulation). In this setting, standard CAPD, which utilizes prolonged dwell times, might not produce sufficient fluid or solute removal. This would necessitate the more frequent use of hypertonic dialysate (2.5 or 4.25 percent dextrose), potentially inducing hyperglycemia, hypertriglyceridemia, and/or weight gain from the increase in glucose absorption, or icodextrin. A better alternative in many cases is multiple short dwells with standard dialysate as with NIPD. The findings are different in "slow" transporters who need long dwell times to adequately remove small solutes. Ultrafiltration is not a problem in this setting, since glucose is also slowly absorbed.

Residual renal function

Patients typically have some residual renal function when they are started on maintenance dialysis. In this setting, it may not be as important to match dwell time with transporter type, since the urine volume can replace the need for ultrafiltration and the minimal renal solute excretion augments that due to dialysis. However, as the residual renal function gradually decreases over time, matching of dwell time to transport type becomes increasingly important [15]. The associated fall in solute clearance can usually be reversed by increasing the dialysis prescription via an increase in the dwell volume or the number of exchanges per day. Either of these modalities will raise the net dialysate flow rate, thereby enhancing the clearance of urea and other small solutes by maintaining a favorable concentration gradient for solute diffusion

Personal issue

Sometimes the choice of PD type is based upon lifestyle or personal issues (such as the desire to work, wish to not do any exchanges during the day, or, in a patient who is not able to do the exchanges themselves). In a prospective randomized study, CCPD provided significantly more time for work, family, and social activities than CAPD [16]. Sleep apnea may also be more responsive to nocturnal PD [17]. In general, automated peritoneal dialysis is superior to CAPD in optimizing fluid and small solute removal in some patients [18]. This is because automated techniques can combine larger dwell volumes, long nocturnal sessions, and add daytime exchanges, thereby moderately increasing solute and fluid removal.

Body surface area — In addition to transport type, residual renal function, and life style choice, another factor to consider when prescribing PD is body surface area because both Kt/V and the weekly creatinine clearance must be normalized to body size. For example, an absolute creatinine clearance of 60 L/week represents different degrees of dialytic solute removal in small versus large patients. Large patients typically need high dialysate volumes, particularly if they are slow transporters and have no residual renal function. With CAPD, the dwell volume is typically 2.5 or 3 liters and some patients require five exchanges per day. With CCPD, the patient will often need 12 to 14 hours of dwell time while on the cycler, using large instilled volumes of dialysate; an alternative is a shorter cycler time (nine to 11 hours) plus one or two daytime exchanges.

A large instilled volume is also required during the daytime dwell and some patients need to perform one manual CAPD exchange to meet the goal for solute clearance. However, increasing the nightly dialysate flow may be superior to adding a manual daytime exchange [19].

Procedures

The main function of a peritoneal dialysis catheter is to permit consistent bidirectional flow of dialysate without extraordinary effort or undue discomfort [20]. The catheter's function depends upon its design, implantation site, and the configuration of the system used to perform dialysis exchanges.

Most catheters are flexible tubes with multiple ports in the distal (intraabdominal) segment which is ideally positioned freely in the intraabdominal pelvic area. The catheter's midportion is normally implanted within the wall of the abdomen via one to two Dacron velour cuffs. With double-cuffed catheters, the deep cuff is imbedded in the abdominal rectus muscle; the superficial cuff in both double cuff and single cuff catheters is placed subcutaneously approximately 2 cm from the catheter exit site on the abdominal wall. Many types of catheters are available for chronic peritoneal dialysis: double cuff straight Tenckhoff catheter, a silicone catheter with a straight (as opposed to coiled) intraabdominal portion is a commonly used catheter [21-23]. The Missouri Swan Neck catheter and the Toronto Western catheter have also been used extensively [24]. Regardless of type, overall catheter survival is approximately 88 percent at one year with removal rates of 15 percent per year [23-25].

The benefit of one catheter over another has not been conclusively demonstrated by prospective, randomized trials [24-26]. A systematic review found no difference related to prevention of peritonitis with respect to straight versus coiled or single versus doubled cuffed catheters, although all cause mortality may be lower with straight catheters (RR of 0.26, 95% CI of 0.07 to 0.99) [27]. A randomized prospective study of 132 patients found no difference in time to catheter malposition, catheter-associated infections, or overall catheter survival [28]. However, an unexplained finding on secondary outcome analysis in this study was that a significantly decreased time to technique failure was observed with the coiled catheter (1.4 versus 2.1 years). This was principally due to inadequate small-solute clearance.

However, the authors report no difference in dialysis adequacy measures between the two groups, suggesting that study bias is responsible for the observed difference. Additional study is needed before one catheter can be recommended over another.

A catheter design in which the "tip" is weighted (ie, self-locating catheter) may reduce the incidence of catheter migration and other complications [29,30]. In a study of 15 and 13 patients with weighted and conventional catheters, respectively, the number of migrating catheters was significantly higher among the conventional group (four versus zero), suggesting that weighted tip catheters may possibly lower the frequency of dialysate flow problems [29]. In a second study, this design was associated with decreased transfers to hemodialysis, and rates of peritonitis, exit site infections, cuff extrusions, obstruction, migration, and leak [30].

Obesity, the presence of stomas, floppy abdominal skin folds, or incontinence of urine or feces are all indications to use an extended catheter system providing a remote exit site location to the upper abdomen or chest, such as the presternal catheter [31]. However, neither catheter was suitable for 25 percent of patients, a finding that emphasizes the benefits of extended catheter systems, such as presternally-located catheters to achieve ideal pelvic positioning of the catheter tip in some patients. Thus, using a single, preferred catheter for all patients may not be the optimal strategy; preoperative evaluation of patients may include assessment of body habitus and consideration of the most appropriate catheter. The catheter used by a PD program primarily depends upon the preferences and experience of the clinician inserting the catheters, with 2005 guidelines stating that no particular catheter is definitively better than the standard silicone Teckhoff catheter for the prevention of peritonitis [32]. Following Crabtree's guidelines, the patient's belt line location should be marked (with the patient clothed) followed by determination of the catheter insertion site, which will suggest the appropriate catheter type [31]. With the patient in the supine position, the position of the deep cuff location, which corresponds to the insertion site, is established by aligning the upper border of the catheter coil with the upper border of the symphysis pubis (a reliable landmark for the ideal position of the catheter tip in the true pelvis). Once the insertion site and deep cuff location are determined, the appropriate catheter can be selected to produce a downwardly-directed tunnel and acceptable exit site location for the patient [31].

Various factors require consideration when inserting a peritoneal dialysis catheter. These include the location of the exit site, use of prophylactic antibiotics, implantation technique, pre- and postoperative care of the catheter, and temporal needs for dialysis [33].

Exit site location

Most PD catheters are placed in a paramedian or lateral abdominal location rather than in the midline. This location allows for positioning of the catheter's deep cuff in or below the rectus muscle, thereby permitting better tissue ingrowth around the cuff due to the richer vascularization of muscle tissue. A paramedian location also provides better structural support for and a strong seal around the catheter, thereby minimizing the risk of peritoneal leak [20-21]. The incidence of peritonitis or exit-site/tunnel infections appears to be similar with midline or lateral insertions [25]. PD catheters can also be placed in a presternal location [34-35]. This location may be desirable in obese patients, very young children (whose need for diapers may contribute to high infection rates with abdominally located PD catheters), patients with ureterocutaneostomies, and those with recurrent exit site infections with abdominal PD catheters [34-35]. Exit site location of a presternal catheter should be at least 3 cm off the midline, and the catheter tubing should not cross the midline of the chest in case cardiac surgery is required [31].

Patient comfort and accessibility to the catheter are also concerns when considering the exit site location. It is therefore best to avoid exit sites over scars, belt lines, and skin folds. To determine the best location, it is often necessary to mark the desired location for the catheter's exit site with the patient in a sitting position (rather than when the patient is lying on the procedure table awaiting catheter insertion).

Exit site size

A nonrandomized prospective study comparing the procedure used to exit the newly-placed catheter from the skin found that the risks of first exit site and tunnel infections, catheter-related peritonitis, and catheter removal were associated with large exit site wounds [36]. Gentle dissection and careful exit-site construction resulting in the smallest possible hole for the exiting catheter is therefore desirable.

Sutures should never be placed at the catheter exit site. Suture material may act as a nidus for bacterial growth and increase the risk of catheter-related infection. Fibroblast ingrowth of the Dacron cuff is sufficient to anchor the catheter, obviating the need for suture material at the exit site.

Antibiotic prophylaxis

There is a paucity of data relating to the efficacy of prophylactic antibiotics before PD catheter implantation. In the largest prospective study, 221 patients undergoing PD catheter placement were randomly assigned to vancomycin (1 gm given intravenously 12 hours prior to the procedure), cefazolin (1 gm given intravenously 3 hours prior to placement), or no antibiotics [37]. At two weeks, the incidence of peritonitis was significantly lower in those given antibiotics, particularly vancomycin (1, 7, and 12 percent for the vancomycin, cefazolin, and no treatment groups, respectively). In a systematic review with analysis of four randomized prospective studies consisting of 335 patients (including the study just mentioned) found that the use of perioperative intravenous antibiotics, compared with no treatment, significantly reduced the risk of peritonitis within one month of surgery (RR of 0.35, 95% CI 0.15 to 0.80) [38]. However, because rise of the incidence of vancomycin resistant Enterococcus sp, the routine use of vancomycin for prophylaxis prior to catheter insertion is not recommended. Other antibiotics, such as a cephalosporin, should therefore be the first choice [39].

Implantation technique

The technique used by a PD program depends upon the preferences and expertise of the surgeon or nephrologist inserting the catheter. Each method of insertion has its benefits and proponents, but no technique has been shown to be preferable overall.

Compared with an upwardly or horizontally-directed PD catheter tunnel, a downwardly-directed tunnel is preferred and recommended by International Guidelines since it may be associated with fewer catheter infections and fewer peritonitis episodes resulting from catheter or tunnel infections [40]. There are several basic methods of PD catheter insertion [20, 21, 34, 41-43]: At the bedside, using a trocar and guidewire technique (generally reserved for temporary acute PD), via laparoscopy, via fluoroscopy, via surgery, either by a standard dissection or by a modification, such as the buried technique (Moncrief-Popovich) or using a presternally-located catheter.

Bedside catheter placement: The benefits of bedside catheter placement are that the technique requires a small incision, is quick and inexpensive, and permits immediate use. The shortcomings are primarily technical: it is a blind procedure, thereby resulting in a greater risk of inadvertent organ and/or vessel perforation; leaks and poor catheter flow are also common.

The problems with this type of catheter placement generally outweigh the advantages in most patients; exceptions include some cases of acute renal failure expected to reverse quickly, and some individuals unable to tolerate the anesthesia required for catheter placement in the operating room. This method is seldom used for chronic catheter placement.

Peritoneoscopy/laparoscopy — Peritoneoscopic catheter placement permits immediate use and, in experienced hands, is a relatively simple and quick procedure [41,42,44]. At one center, a significantly lower incidence of flow dysfunction was observed with such placement (particularly advanced laparoscopic techniques) compared with an open surgical procedure [42]. Video-assisted laparoscopic procedures constitute an effective means for managing several problems related to peritoneal dialysis such as catheter malfunction, preimplantation evaluation, location of the source of the dialysate leak, and assessment of the causes for peritonitis [45].

Fluoroscopy — Percutaneous fluoroscopy-guided placement provides accurate placement with little waiting time and a relatively small incision [43]. Limited data suggest that this approach provides similar outcomes compared with more invasive techniques [43]; however, the incidence of late leakage appears to be increased.

Surgery — Surgical placement of catheters has the advantage of precise catheter placement with little risk of viscus perforation. Disadvantages are the longer time involved (including operating room scheduling), greater cost, and larger incision required. The buried catheter technique differs from the standard surgical technique in that the entire catheter remains buried subcutaneously until it is ready to be used, usually four to six weeks after catheter placement. At that time, the catheter is exteriorized. This method was developed to possibly reduce peritonitis and catheter infections by allowing complete sinus tract healing and fibroblast ingrowth into the cuff before local trauma to the exit site could occur. However, randomized prospective trials comparing this method with the standard surgical technique showed conflicting results [46-48]. Most programs continue to use the standard technique unless early infection rates are high. The principal disadvantages of the buried technique are the need for two procedures and the longer waiting time for catheter use.

A Prospective randomized study comparing the open surgery with laparoscopic-assisted placement of Tenckhoff peritoneal dialysis catheter found that laparoscopic assisted percutaneous puncture exhibited no superiority to open surgery. The laparoscopy had a longer operative time (68.32+/-31.90 versus 46.68+/-15.99 min; P<0.001), shorter wound length (1.69+/-0.46 versus 2.34+/-0.84 cm; P<0.001), and higher costs (P<0.001) compared with open surgery. Laparoscopy tended to have a higher incidence of pericannular bleeding (21.6% versus 7.5%) and a lower rate of early catheter migration (2.7% versus 15.0%), but its early/late/overall complication rate did not statistically differ. No surgical mortality occurred. Rate and cause of overall mortality or catheter dropout did not statistically differ. Catheter longevity was equivalent in both groups. The authors concluded that the open surgery demand shorter operative time and the reduced equipment requirement can increase cost-effectiveness [49]. However, a survey of surgical residency program directors showed that, although most programs included peritoneal dialysis catheter placement as a procedure taught to their trainees, most surgeons placed two or fewer than five catheters during their training [50]. Thus, experience in individual programs will dictate the technique and operators placing PD catheters.

Postoperative catheter care: Catheter patency should always be assured before leaving the operating room by infusing one liter of peritoneal dialysate over five minutes and allowing an additional five minutes for drainage, or by instilling and aspirating saline [21]. Newly placed catheters are usually flushed with small volumes of dialysate (heparin may be added as 500 to 1000 units/L dialysate if fibrin or clots are evident) until the effluent is clear. The catheter is then capped and a dressing applied to the site. There are few controlled trials of optimal catheter care post-placement, but most suggest that the catheter site be covered with gauze dressing and remain undisturbed for several days [21]. The catheter should be immobilized with a dressing and/or tape to minimize trauma [21]. Infrequent dressing changes (eg, once/week) are probably sufficient for the first one to two weeks after implantation.

It is important to minimize catheter movement and handling, since local trauma can increase the risk of bacterial colonization with subsequent infection. To minimize the risk of fluid leak, it is preferable to wait at least 10 to 14 days after catheter insertion before beginning peritoneal dialysis. If PD is required less than 10 days following catheter placement, small volume exchanges (ie, less than 1500 mL) performed in the recumbent position only (eg, with a cycler or chronic ambulatory peritoneal dialysis with supine dwells only) can be performed with little risk of leak [22, 51]. Some may choose to "lock" the PD catheter during temporary cessation of PD in an attempt to avoid clotting of the PD catheter. Heparin can be used for this purpose in the same dosages used to lock hemodialysis catheters, as the heparin is not peritoneally absorbed. Others may elect not to lock the PD catheter as the risk of catheter occlusion during non-use is probably low.

Exit site care: The International Society for Peritoneal Dialysis published guidelines for practices relating to the exit-site of peritoneal catheters [28, 32]. After placement of the catheter, dressing changes are not needed until about 7 to 10 days post-operatively. If dressing changes are done, a peritoneal dialysis nurse should perform sterile dressing changes until the patient is trained and the exit site is well-healed. The site should be dry until it is well-healed, which precludes taking showers or baths, usually for a period of up to two weeks. For chronic care, Exit sites should be washed daily or every other day with antibacterial soap or an antiseptic (either povidone iodine or chlorhexidine). Cleansers may be individualized based upon allergies and should not be transferred to other containers because of the risk of contamination. Cleansers that are toxic to cells or the normal granulation tissue of the exit site, such as hydrogen, which is drying, should be avoided for routine care.

RISK FACTORS

A major challenge to the growth of PD, and home dialysis in general, is the fact that the majority of dialysis patients in many regions are elderly and have barriers to self-care [52]. Impediments for a proper self-care were decreased muscle strengths, decreased manual dexterity, decreased vision or hearing, immobility, poor health/frailty, poor hygiene, cognitive or language barriers, history of non-compliance, psychiatric condition and dementia or poor memory function [53]. Decreased strength to lift PD bags was present in 37% of a dialysis population (median age of 73years), while decreased vision, decreased hearing and immobility were present in 25%, 17% and 20% of the population, respectively[54]. Thus, support by family members may be required for many patients to perform PD.

In a large prospective assessment of consecutive incident ESRD patients found that patients with barriers were older, weighed less and were more likely to be female, start dialysis as an inpatient and have a history of vascular disease, cardiac disease and cancer. Family support was associated with an increase in PD eligibility from 63% to 80% (P = 0.003) and PD choice from 40% to 57% (P = 0.03) in patients with barriers to self-care. Family support increased incidence PD utilization from 23% to 39% among patients with barriers to self-care (P = 0.009). When family support was available, 34% received family-assisted PD, 47% received home care assisted PD, 12% received both family- and home care-assisted PD, and 7% performed only self-care PD [55].

Other medical conditions predisposing to risk of PD include obesity, abdominal scarring, ascites, diverticulitis, abdominal hernia, inflammatory bowel disease, ileo-colostomy, abdominal aortic aneurysm, previous major abdominal surgery, bowel cancer, percutaneous gastric tube, ileal conduit, polycystic kidneys and ischaemic gut. [55-57]. Contraindications, barriers to self-care, availability of family support and the social conditions should be considered before PD utilization.

References

[1] Twardowski ZJ. Peritoneal dialysis

[2] Teitelbaum I, Burkart J. Peritoneal dialysis

[3] Dell'Aquila R, Rodighiero MP, Spanó E, et al. Advances in the technology

[4] Juergensen PH, Murphy AL, Pherson KA, et al. Tidal peritoneal dialysis

[5] Juergensen PH, Murphy AL, Pherson KA, et al. Tidal peritoneal dialysis

[6] European Best Practice Guidelines for peritoneal dialysis. Nephrol Dial Transplant 2005; 20(Suppl 9):3.

[7] Diaz-Buxo JA. Evolution of continuous flow peritoneal dialysis

[8] Freida P, Issad B. Continuous flow peritoneal dialysis

[9] Rabindranath KS, Adams J, Ali TZ, et al. Continuous ambulatory peritoneal dialysis

[10] Rabindranath KS, Adams J, Ali TZ, et al. Automated vs continuous ambulatory peritoneal dialysis

[11] Michels WM, Verduijn M, Boeschoten EW, et al. Similar survival

[12] Mehrotra R, Chiu YW, Kalantar-Zadeh K, Vonesh E. The outcomes of continuous ambulatory and automated peritoneal dialysis

[13] Twardowski, ZJ. PET—A simpler approach. In: Advances in Peritoneal Dialysis, vol. 7, Khanna, R, et al (Eds), Peritoneal Dialysis Bulletin, Nashville, 1990, pp. 186-191.

[14] Twardowski ZJ. Nightly peritoneal dialysis

[15] Davies SJ, Phillips L, Griffiths AM, et al. What really happens to people on long-term peritoneal dialysis

[16] Bro S, Bjorner JB, Tofte-Jensen P, et al. A prospective, randomized multicenter study comparing APD and CAPD treatment
[17] Tang SC, Lam B, Ku PP, et al. Alleviation of sleep apnea
[18] Pérez-Fontán M, Rodríguez-Carmona A. Comparing CAPD and automated peritoneal dialysis
[19] Demetriou D, Habicht A, Schillinger M, et al. Adequacy of automated peritoneal dialysis
[20] Lee HB, Park MS, Cha MK, et al. The peritoneal access
[21] Gokal R, Alexander S, Ash S, et al. Peritoneal catheters and exit-site practices toward optimum peritoneal access
[22] Teitelbaum I, Burkart J. Peritoneal dialysis
[23] Piraino B. Which catheter
[24] Eklund BH, Honkanen EO, Kala AR, Kyllönen LE. Peritoneal dialysis
[25] Strippoli GF, Tong A, Johnson D, et al. Catheter-related interventions to prevent peritonitis
[26] Stegmayr BG, Wikdahl AM, Bergström M, et al. A randomized clinical trial
[27] Crabtree JH, Burchette RJ. Prospective comparison of downward and lateral peritoneal dialysis
[28] Johnson DW, Wong J, Wiggins KJ, et al. A randomized controlled trial
[29] Cavagna R, Tessarin C, Tarroni G, et al. The self-locating catheter
[30] Di Paolo N, Capotondo L, Sansoni E, et al. The self-locating catheter
[31] Crabtree, JH. Selected best demonstrated practices in peritoneal dialysis access. Kidney Int 2006; 70:S27.
[32] Piraino B, Bailie GR, Bernardini J, et al. Peritoneal dialysis
[33] Ash SR. Chronic peritoneal dialysis
[34] Twardowski ZJ, Prowant BF, Pickett B, et al. Four-year experience with swan neck presternal peritoneal dialysis
[35] Warchol S, Roszkowska-Blaim M, Sieniawska M. Swan neck presternal peritoneal dialysis
[36] Crabtree JH, Fishman A, Siddiqi RA, Hadnott LL. The risk
[37] Gadallah MF, Ramdeen G, Mignone J, et al. Role of preoperative antibiotic
[38] Strippoli GF, Tong A, Johnson D, et al. Antimicrobial agents to prevent peritonitis
[39] Keane WF, Alexander SR, Bailie GR, et al. Peritoneal dialysis
[40] Golper TA, Brier ME, Bunke M, et al. Risk factors for peritonitis
[41] Copley JB, Lindberg JS, Back SN, Tapia NP. Peritoneoscopic placement of Swan neck peritoneal dialysis

[42] Crabtree JH, Fishman A. A laparoscopic method for optimal peritoneal dialysis
[43] Moon
[44] Wright MJ, Bel'eed K, Johnson BF, et al. Randomized prospective comparison of laparoscopic and open peritoneal dialysis
[45] Jwo SC, Chen KS, Lin YY. Video-assisted laparoscopic procedures in peritoneal dialysis. Surg Endosc 2003;17:1666-70.
[46] Danielsson A, Blohmé L, Tranaeus A, Hylander B. A prospective randomized study of the effect of a subcutaneously "buried" peritoneal dialysis
[47] Wu CC, Su PF, Chiang SS
[48] Brown PA, McCormick BB, Knoll G, et al. Complications and catheter
[49] Jwo SC, Chen KS, Lee CC, Chen HY. Prospective randomized study for comparison of open surgery with laparoscopic-assisted placement of Tenckhoff peritoneal dialysis catheter--a single center experience and literature review. J Surg Res 2010;159:489-96.
[50] Wong LP, Liebman SE, Wakefield KA, Messing S. Training of surgeons in peritoneal dialysis
[51] European Best Practice Guidelines for peritoneal dialysis. Nephrol Dial Transplant 2005; 20(Suppl 9):3.
[52] Burkart J: Role of peritoneal dialysis in the era of the resurgence of home hemodialysis. Hemodial Int 2008; Suppl 1: S51-54.
[53] Chaudhary K, Sangha H and Khanna R: Peritoneal dialysis first: rationale. Clin J Am Soc Nephrol 2011; 6: 447-456.
[54] Lameire N and Van Biesen W: Epidemiology of peritoneal dialysis: a story of believers and nonbelievers. Nat Rev Nephrol 2010; 6: 75-82.
[55] Oliver MJ, Garg AX, Blake PG, et al.: Impact of contraindications, barriers to self-care and support on incident peritoneal dialysis utilization. Nephrology Dialysis Transplantation 2010; 25: 2737-2744.
[56] Stuart S, Booth TC, Cash CJ, et al.: Complications of continuous ambulatory peritoneal dialysis. Radiographics 2009; 29: 441-460.
[57] Liakopoulos V and Dombros N: Patient selection for automated peritoneal dialysis: for whom, when? Perit Dial Int 2009; 29 Suppl 2: S102-107.

In: Peritoneal Dialysis
Editors: A. Agarwal, L. Salman et al.
ISBN: 978-1-62257-896-2

Chapter 2

ADVANCES IN PERITONEAL DIALYSIS

Aamir Jalal Al Mosawi*
[1] University Hospital in Al Kadhimiyia, Baghdad Iraq
[2] Training and Development Center, Iraqi Ministry of Health, Iraq

ABSTRACT

Peritoneal dialysis (PD) enjoyed huge growth in the 1980s, followed by a rapid decline in the late 1990s, and a now persistently low utilization rate in many countries, including the United States. Recent clinical research data indicate a survival advantage for patients started on PD. Residual renal function is better preserved with PD.

New peritoneal dialysis (PD) patients have a better survival than new hemodialysis (HD) patients in the first year on dialysis. During long-term treatment, this changes into a survival advantage for HD. The superior initial survival on PD is thought to be related to a better preservation of residual renal function of PD patients compared to HD. The magnitude of the residual glomerular filtration rate (rGFR) in PD patients is not only associated with better survival, but also with less uremic symptoms, such as loss of appetite, and also with higher scores on quality of life tests. Adequacy targets are being revised and will likely allow PD prescriptions to be simplified. The physiology of the peritoneum is better understood and treatment strategies reflect that understanding. New solutions have

* E-mail address: almosawiAJ@yahoo.com

been developed in response to studies that have assessed the impact of conventional PD dialysate on the structure and function of the peritoneum.

Despite technology advances, prevention of peritonitis remains one of the major challenges in peritoneal dialysis (PD). Several innovative developments have shown an impact on peritonitis rates. Innovative antimicrobial-coated catheter modifications have been introduced, showing promising results in vitro. Topical application of antimicrobial agents such as mupirocin to prevent exit-site infections has been successfully used. New alternative agents for topical exit-site care with reduced potential for antimicrobial resistance are under development. Flushing before fill and avoidance of spiking of solution bags has improved peritonitis rates, as have innovative connectology and double-bag systems. The incidence of peritonitis has markedly improved since the end of the 1980s, but infection remains a significant complication of chronic PD. Quantifying the role of the many practices and devices in reducing complications is difficult, but their combined effect has clearly improved peritonitis outcomes.

The objective of modern PD is to extend its initial survival advantage to long-term treatment. Recent advances in knowledge of mechanisms and new dialysis solutions are likely to make this possible. Technologic advances in PD could have an important impact on patient care.

Advances in Peritoneal Dialysis: Historic Background

The Early Concepts of Peritoneal Dialysis

The earliest concept of peritoneal dialysis emerged in the early 1740's with the work of Stephen Hales and Christopher Warrick. Stephen Hales and Christopher Warrick, an English surgeon, laid the cornerstone for peritoneal dialysis in humans in 1744: they attempted to treat a 50-year-old patient with ascites by first removing the excess abdominal fluid from the woman before using a leather tube to infuse a solution consisting of 50% water and 50% wine into her abdomen. [1]. Friedrich Daniel Von Recklinghaussen was the first to describe the gross and cellular anatomy of the peritoneum in 1862 [2, 3, 4].

G. Wegner, in Germany, determined the absorption rate of various solutions from the peritoneum as early as 1877. G. Wegner described the basis for using the peritoneum for fluid removal, or peritoneal ultrafiltration. Wegner performed the first animal experiments to observe the metabolic transport processes occurring through the peritoneum. He injected solutions of various contents and temperatures into rabbits and discovered that a concentrated sugar solution would lead to an increased amount of fluid in the abdominal cavity. Wegner also described the effects of changes in body temperature occurring after intraperitoneal infusion of solutions with various temperatures and also reported the effects of concentrated dextrose or glycerin solutions on the volume of outflow obtained in the peritoneal effluent, perhaps the first evidence of osmotic ultrafiltration (UF) [5,6].

In 1894, two Englishmen, Ernest Henry Starling and Alfred Herbert Tubby, first described the fluid removal characteristics of the peritoneum and discovered that fluid removal through the peritoneum was effected by blood vessels in the membrane. They studied the bidirectional transfer of molecules across the peritoneal and pleural membranes and demonstrated the rapid absorption of isotonic solutions and slow absorption of serum [7, 8].

By 1920, it had been recognized that, regardless of the infusate osmolality, the fluid was completely absorbed within 20 hours of infusion [9, 10, 11]. These observations led to the administration of intraperitoneal fluids to infants with severe dehydration when the oral route was not possible [12, 13]. This may have been the first therapeutic use of the peritoneal membrane.

The first quarter of the 20th century established the physiologic milestones for peritoneal dialysis (PD) with emphasis on the relationship between osmolality of the fluids and peritoneal ultrafiltration and absorption [10, 14], and the bidirectional flux of small molecules between the peritoneal cavity and the intravascular compartment. The contributions of WN Orlow, Clark, Putnam, and others confirmed the peritoneal membrane permeability for sodium and other minerals [15, 16, 17, 18, 19]. In 1895, WN Orlow pointed out that fluid absorption occurs from the peritoneal cavity [20].

The concept of osmotic equilibrium between peritoneal fluid and plasma was established by Putnam in 1922, who concluded that mass transfer was driven by passive concentration gradients rather than active membrane transport [16].

Klapp first observed that heat applied to the anterior abdominal wall could accelerate the exchange of substances between the ip cavity and the blood compartment [18]. This observation was a precursor of the concept of augmentation dialysis. Clark confirmed these findings twenty years later by using ip infusions of warm solutions and suggested that vasodilatation was responsible for the accelerated rate of exchange [19].The initial uremic models consisted of rabbits and guinea pigs subjected to ureteral ligation. Intraperitoneal exchanges lasting 2 to 4 hours were utilized. Although there was moderate absorption of the dialysate due to its hypotonicity relative to uremic plasma, definite clinical improvement was noted in the animals after dialysis.

In 1918, Desider Engel, working first in Prague and then in China, demonstrated that protein can pass through the peritoneal membrane [21]. This significant finding was applied by later investigators in their efforts to show that peritoneal dialysis may be more efficient in removing large molecules. In 1919. M. Rosenberg noted that the same fluid in the peritoneum contained the same amount of urea that is found in the blood, indicating that urea could, in fact, be removed using peritoneal dialysis [22].In 1923 that Tracy Putnam, at Johns Hopkins University, suggested that the peritoneum might be used to correct psychological problems [23].

The First Human Peritoneal Dialysis

George Ganter suggested the use of the peritoneum as a large endogenous dialysis membrane. In 1923, in experiments on ureter-ligated guinea pigs and rabbits, he demonstrated that the single or repeated instillation (after effective draining) of physiological NaCl solution improves both the symptoms of uremia and the blood urea nitrogen level.

The first peritoneal dialysis for uremic patients was performed at the University of Würzburg by George Ganter. In 1923, after having experimented on animals, Ganter used a sterile physiological solution that contained the proper amount of electrolytes with dextrose added for fluid removal. The solution was placed in large bottles that were then boiled to insure that the bacteria had been killed. The solution was instilled into the patient's peritoneum through a simple hollow needle, with rubber tubing serving as the conduit between the bottle and the needle [24, 25].

In the early 1920's, Stephen Rosenak and P. Sewon, working in Europe, developed a metal catheter for continuous lavage of the peritoneum that helped overcome some of the problems with access [26].

Between 1924 and 1938, several medical teams in the United States and Germany performed regularly repeated (intermittent) PD treatment and used the procedure for the short-term of chronic renal failure [25].Intermittent PD never became popular for management of chronic kidney failure because of the risk of underdialysis, malnutrition, and frequent episodes of peritonitis. [27]. However, some dedicated units achieved good results [28].

Continuous Peritoneal Dialysis

The development of continuous peritoneal dialysis occurred at Wisconsin General Hospital in 1936. J. B. Wear, I. R. Sisk, and A. J. Tinkle used peritoneal dialysis on a patient who was suffering from urinary obstruction [29]. They were able to maintain the patient on continuous dialysis until the obstruction was resolved, demonstrating for the first time that a patient could be safely treated with continued peritoneal dialysis.

P.S.M. Kop was an associate of Willem Kolff's in Netherlands during the mid-1940's.Kop developed an integrated system that used gravity as the means to instill the dialysis solution into the peritoneal cavity. The components of Kop's system could be easily sterilized; porcelain containers to hold the solution, latex rubber tubing to carry the solution down to the patient, and a large glass catheter to instill the solution into the patient's peritoneal cavity. Kop's group treated 21 patients with success in ten of them [30]. Seligman, Jacob Fine, and Howard Frank modified Kop system to overcome technical problems, such as optimal flow rates and modification of the solution to suit patient needs. They used large bottles of solution that were sterilized o prevent bacterial contamination , and they used two catheters to minimize any potential obstruction during the outflow phase of the procedure[31].In 1945, the Seligman group used their system to treat a patient who was suffering from acute renal failure induced by an overdose of sulfa drugs. The patient's successful recovery was one of the primary milestones in the development of peritoneal dialysis.

Peritoneal Dialysis Catheter

This safe access to the abdomen for peritoneal dialysis is provided by a catheter. Originally, metal cannulae were used to gain access to the abdominal cavity, but were replaced by stomach and oxygen tubes later on. In 1952, Arthur Grollman working in Southwestern Medical School of Dallas developed a catheter that would make peritoneal dialysis treatments accessible for patients with chronic kidney failure. Grollman used a one liter container with a cap to which a plastic tube was attached. The flexible catheter with very small holes in the distal end prevented the patient's body tissue from impeding the drainage; the result was better inflow and outflow of the fluid .Grollman suggested that the fluid be instilled by gravity and that it should dwell for 30 minutes, at which time it would be drained out into the same container. He suggested that the technique be repeated on an hourly basis until the patient's chemistries returned to normal. Grollman was the first to describe the intermittent method of peritoneal dialysis that we use today [32]. In 1959 Morton Maxwell designed PD system that requires fewer connections and disconnections. Maxwell technique was quite simple; instill 2 liters of peritoneal solution into the peritoneum; let it dwell for 30 minutes; then drain the fluid into the original bottles. The procedure was continued until the patient's blood chemistries were normal. Maxwell performed a number of successful peritoneal dialyses using this method [33].

Paul Doolan developed a catheter for long-term use in 1959. It was made of polyethylene with a unique geometry of holes to prevent clogging, while maximizing the flow rate. The flexible catheter contained a number of grooved segments to prevent blockage of drain holes and maximizing drainage. In 1956 Richard Ruben, performed the first peritoneal dialysis over a period of seven months, using the Doolan catheter as well as a permanent catheter that could remain in the abdominal cavity. [34].

Automated Peritoneal Dialysis Machine

Automated peritoneal dialysis was introduced in 1962 by Fred Boen of Washington University. The automated unit could be operated unattended during the night. The machine required a 40-liter container of PD solution. Boen method significantly cut the amount of time needed to open and close the tubing system and connect or disconnect bags, as required by manual CAPD. Full containers were delivered to the patients' homes and retrieved when empty. Intermittent peritoneal dialysis was performed weekly. Boen also developed an automatic solenoid device that would open and close a switch to meter the fluid in and out of the peritoneum.

Boen used a permanently indwelling peritoneal access tube into which a long catheter that could be inserted and removed. After each treatment, the catheter was removed and indwelling tube was capped. This open system was quite vulnerable to peritonitis, forcing Boen to abandon the technique. He then turned to an intermittent method in which a new catheter was placed into the peritoneum before each procedure and removed on completion of the treatment. Boen used intermittent technique for home use. A physician would go to the patient's house, insert the catheter, begin the exchange, and then leave after the procedure had begun. On completion of the treatment, which would last for about 24 hours, the patient's caregiver would shut down the machine and help the patient remove the catheter. The wound would be covered with a bandage, and the patient would lead a normal life until the next weekend when dialysis would be preformed again. Although the dialysis procedure itself became quite routine, the logistical support required prevented widespread use of the technique [35, 36].

In 1963, Henry Tenckhoff of Washington University designed a simplified delivery system to avoid the need to transport the 40-liter bottles. By instilling water still in the patient's house to provide sterile water. The water was mixed with a peritoneal concentrate to provide the proper dialyzing fluid. Tenckhoff's group also developed a solenoid system that would automatically fill and empty the peritoneum. The system worked, but it remained cumbersome and time consuming and, in some cases, it was dangerous because of the high pressures involved in the use of the still.

In 1968 Henry Tenckhoff developed the catheter named after him. Up until then, the widely used stylet catheter had already made it possible to treat patients with chronic renal failure using peritoneal disease. However, the "repeated puncture technique" meant placing a new catheter in the abdominal cavity for each treatment. This time-consuming procedure bothered both medical personnel and patients. The Tenckhoff catheter is still in use today. Made from silicone, it has one or two cuffs which help the catheter to grow into the peritoneum as well as into deeper layers of connective tissue.

In 1969, Tenckhoff's group used an inline "reverse osmosis" (R/O) water purification system to avoid the need for the large bottles and the still [37]. The R/O water was mixed with the peritoneal concentrate, and an integrated solenoid controller related the inflow and outflow of the peritoneal solution. Tenckhoff integrated the R/O system into a simplified automatic peritoneal dialysis machine that could be operated easily and effectively by the patient at home. The system became the prototype for all the R/O peritoneal machines that were developed later.

Permanent Catheter

Russell Palmer and Wayne Quinton in 1962 developed a silicone catheter that could be left in the abdomen permanently. The catheter was sealed properly at the exit site and prevented bacteria from migrating to the peritoneal cavity. The development of permanent catheter was a significant step forward in the development of chronic peritoneal dialysis because it provided continuous access to the peritoneum for the first time [38].

Tenckhoff modified Palmers catheter so that it would be easier to insert and use [39] He shortened the catheter and suggested two designs, straight and curled. In addition, he added Dacron felt cuffs to help seal the openings through the peritoneum .He also developed an insertion tool, called a trocar, which was designed to provide easy placement of the catheter. Tenckhoff now had a complete system for doing chronic intermittent peritoneal dialysis.

Cycler Development

Norman Lasker's and Mark Schachter (an engineer with the Gottscho Packaging Equipment Co.,) designed a mechanical system for peritoneal dialysis. The system which was designed to use 2- liter bottles and flexible plastic reservoir bags, was safe, easy to set up, and easy to operate. Two important features included in the system were the ability to measure the volume of fluid to be instilled into the peritoneal cavity and the ability to warm the solution before the "fill" cycle. Lasker called his system the "peritoneal cycler"[40].

Continuous Ambulatory Peritoneal Dialysis (CAPD)

The advent of continuous ambulatory peritoneal dialysis (CAPD) in the late 1970s has dramatically changed treatment options available to the patient with ESRD. Since it was approved for reimbursement in the States by Medicare in 1979, the use of CAPD has increased rapidly, and, by 1983, an estimated 8,000 patients, two-thirds of patients on home dialysis, or 12% of the entire chronic dialysis population were being treated by this modality. Diffusion has resulted from a combination of strong professional endorsement, patient acceptance, and vigorous marketing efforts by industrial producers of CAPD supplies and equipment.

CAPD probably originated in Austin, Texas, in 1978. Robert Popovich (a biomedical engineer at the University of Texas) and Jack Moncrief were the first to describe CAPD. They developed comprehensive calculations based on the amount and dwell time of the dialysis solution, and determined the effective removal of uremic toxins. Robert Popovich and his associates determined that five exchanges of 2 liters per day would achieve the appropriate chemistries, and that they needed to remove 12 liters of equilibrated solution from the patient each day. Jack Moncrief and Robert Popovich used a standard 2-liter bottle and attached a simple piece of tubing to it, along with a Tenckhoff catheter. Fluid was instilled for a period of four hours and then drained out. The procedure, which they called Continuous Ambulatory Peritoneal Dialysis (CAPD), allowed them to control successfully and simply a patient's chemistries and fluid removal. The only shortcomings of the technique were potential complications of infection and protein loss. Moncrief noted that the protein loss was observed very early in the treatment series, and it became evident that the diet of the patient would have to be supplemented with protein, while other dietary restrictions could be relaxed. Once Moncrief determined that the solution could be left in the peritoneum overnight without compromising the patient, a patient (Peter Pilcher) was trained to do the exchanges by himself. He dialyzed using CAPD for more than two months and then received a kidney transplant [41, 42].

Until 1978, peritoneal dialysis solution (PD solution) was only available in glass containers, connected to the permanent catheter with plastic tubes. Patients had to attach the tubes to the catheter every time they added or removed solution. Because of the high number of connections and disconnections, the danger of peritoneal infection was always imminent. Dimitrios Oreopoulos from Toronto Western Hospital made CAPD more practical by introducing disposable plastic bags, which lowered the peritonitis rate considerably. Once the dialysis solution was introduced into the abdominal cavity, the plastic bag could be rolled up and remained connected to the patient's body for the duration of the treatment. To remove the solution, the bag was unrolled, and gravity pulled the used dialysis solution into the bag. At the end of the procedure, the bag was removed from the catheter and a fresh bag attached. This new technology offered patients more comfort and relative freedom [43].

Intraperitoneal Insulin Administration

Initially, patients with diabetes were not treated with dialysis because of the risk of exacerbating hyperglycemia. Carl Kjellstrand of Minnesota University suggested the intraperitoneal administration of insulin [44]. In 1979 CT. Flynn's proposed that renal failure patients with diabetes might do better on CAPD. It was Flynn's contention that CAPD's long dwell time for dialysis fluid in the peritoneal cavity made it appropriate as a medium for insulin administration. Because of its large molecular structure (5000MW), insulin is slowly absorbed from the peritoneum. Thus, by incorporating insulin into the CAPD procedure, Flynn was able to maintain blood sugars in the normal range required for good patient management. Currently, more than 30% of the patients on peritoneal dialysis are diabetic. In fact, intraperitoneal insulin administration has become an important technique in treating the diabetic complications of renal disease. [45].

REFERENCES

[1] An eighteenth century suggestion for peritoneal dialysis. An editorial. *Internatl J Artif Organs* 1980, 3(2):67-68.

[2] Cunningham, RS. The physiology of the serous membranes. *Physiol Rev 1926*, 6:242.

[3] von Recklinghaussen, FT. Die Lymphgefässe und ihre Beziehung zum Bindegewebe. Berlin, Germany: Hirshwald; 1862.

[4] von Recklinghaussen FT. Zur fettresorption. Virchows Arch 26:172, 1863

[5] Wegner, G. Chirurgische Bermekungen über die Peritonealhöle, mit besonderer Berucksichtigung der Ovariotomie. *Arch Klin Chir* 1877, 20:51,

[6] Wegner, G. Surgical comments on peritoneal cavity with special emphasis on ovariotomy. *Arch f Klin Chir* v 20:53-145, 1877.

[7] Starling, EH; Tubby, A.H. On the paths of absorption from the peritoneal cavity. *J Physiol* 1894, 16:140.

[8] Starling, EH; Tubby, AH. The influence of mechanical factors on lymph production. *J Physiol* 1894, 16:140 *(London)*

[9] Cunningham RS. Studies on absorption from serous cavities, III. *Am J Physiol*, 1920, 53:488.

[10] Schechter, AJ; Cary MK; Carpentieri AL, et al. Changes in composition of fluids injected into the peritoneal cavity. *Am J Dis Child* 1933, *46:1015.*

[11] Hamburger, HJ. Ueber die Regelung der osmotischen Spannkraft von Flüssigkeiten in Bauch-und Pericardialhöhle. *Archiv f Phys du Bois-Reymond* 1895, 281.

[12] Blackfan, KD; Maxcy, KF. The intraperitoneal injection of saline solution. *Am J Dis Child* 1918, 15:19.

[13] Berg, M. Die Anwendung der intraperitonealen Infusion beim wasserverarmten Saügling. *Ztschr f Kinderheilkunde* 1921, 29:15.

[14] Leathes, JB; Starling, EH. On the absorption of salt solutions from the pleural cavities. *J Physiol* 1895, 18:106,

[15] Orlow, WN. Einige Versuche über die Resorption in der Bauchhöle. *Arch f Phys Pflüger* 1895, 59:170.

[16] Putnam, TJ. The living peritoneum as a dialyzing membrane. *Am J Physiol* 1922, 63:548.

[17] Abbott, WE, Shea, P. The treatment of temporary renal insufficiency by peritoneal lavage. *Am J Med Sci* 1946, 211:312.

[18] Klapp R. Ueber Bauchfelresorption. *Mitt Grenzgeb der Med u Chir* 1902, 10:254.

[19] Clark AJ. Absorption from the peritoneal cavity. *J Pharmacol* 16:415, 1921

[20] Orlow, W. N. Some studies of the absorption of the abdominal cavity. *Arch f Physiol* 1927, 103:423-427.

[21] Engel, D. Uber die ausspulbarkeit von toxin, antikorpern und artfremden eiweis durch des lebende peritoneum. [The rinsability of toxin, antibody and foreign protein through the living peritoneum.] *Centralbl f Bacteriologie* 1927, 103:423-427.

[22] Rosenberg, M. Uber stickstoffhaltiqe retentiosstoffe im blute und in anderen korpeflussigkeiten bei nephritikern. [Nitrogenous retention of substances in blood and in other body fluids in the core of the kidneys.] *Berl Klin Wochenschr* 1923, 53:548-565, 1923

[23] Putnam, T. The living peritoneum as a dialyzing membrane. *Am J Physiol* 1923, 3:548-565.

[24] Ganter, G. About the elimination of poisonous substances from the blood by dialysis. *Munch Med Wchnschr* 1923, 70:1478-1480.

[25] Teschner,M; Heidland,A; Klassen,A; Sebekova,K; BahnerU.Georg Ganter--a pioneer of peritoneal dialysis and his tragic academic demise at the hand of the Nazi regime. J Nephrol. 2004, 17(3):457-60.

[26] Rosenak, S; Siwon, P. Experimentelle untersuchungen uber die peritoneale aussscheidung harnpflichtiger substanzen aus dem blute. [Experimental investigation of the peritoneal clearance of ureabound substances from the blood.] *mitt grenzgeb Med Chir* 1926, 39:391-408.

[27] Krediet, RT. 30 years of peritoneal dialysis development: the past and the future. Perit Dial Int. 2007, 27 Suppl 2:S35-41.

[28] Oreopoulos, DG. Chronic peritoneal dialysis. Clin Nephrol. 1978, 9:165-73.

[29] Wear, JB; Sisk, IR; Trinkle, A. J. Peritoneal levage in the treatment of uremia. *J Urol* 1938, 39:53-62.

[30] Kolff, WJ. New ways to treating uremia. J.A. Churchill Ltd. London, pp. 91-97, 1947.

[31] Frank, H; Seligman. A; Fine, J. Treatment of uremia after acute renal failure by peritoneal irrigation. JAMA 1946, 130:703-705.

[32] Grollman, A; Turner, LB; McLean JA. Intermittent peritoneal lavage in nephrectomized dogs and its application to the human being. *Arch Intern Med* 1951, 87:376-390.

[33] Maxwell, MH; Rockney, RE; Kleeman, CR. Peritoneal dialysis, techniques and application. *JAMA* 1959, 170:917-924.

[34] Doolan, P D; Murphy Jr., W P; Wiggins, RA; et al. An evaluation of intermittent peritoneal lavage. *Am J Med* 1959, 26:831-844.

[35] Boen, ST. *Peritoneal dialysis.* Van Gorcum & Comp N.V. Amsterdam, 26, 1959.

[36] Boen, S T; Mion, C M; Curtis, FK; et al. Periodic peritoneal dialysis using repeated puncture technique and automatic cycling machine. *Trans Am Soc Artif Intern Organs* v 10:409-414, 1964.

[37] 37 Tenckhoff, H; Meston B; Shilipeater G. A simplified automatic peritoneal dialysis system. *Trans Am Soc Artif Intern Organs* 1972, 17:436-439.

[38] Palmer, A; Quinton, W E; Gray, J E. Prolonged peritoneal dialysis for chronic renal failure. *Lancet* 1964 1:700-702.

[39] Tenckhoff, H; Schecter, H. A bacteriologically safe peritoneal access device. *Trans Am Soc Artif Intern Organs* 11968, 4:181-183.

[40] Lasker, N; McCauley, EP; Passarotti, CT. Chronic peritoneal dialysis. *Trans Am Soc Artif Intern Organs* 1966, 12:94-105.

[41] Popovich, RP; Moncrief, JW; Nolph, KD; et al. Continuous ambulatory peritoneal dialysis. *Ann Intern Med* 1978, 88:449.

[42] Popovich, RP; Moncrief, JW; Nolph, KD; et al. Continuous ambulatory peritoneal dialysis. Ann Intern Med. 1978, 88:449-56.

[43] Oreopoulos, DG;Robson, M; Faller, B; Ogilvie, R, et al; Continuous ambulatory peritoneal dialysis: a new era in the treatment of chronic renal failure. Clin Nephrol. 1979, 11:125-8.

[44] Crossley, K; Kjellstrand, CM. Intraperitoneal insuling for control of blood surgar in diabetic patients during peritoneal dialysis. *Br Med J* 1971, 1:269-270,

[45] Flynn, CT; Nanson, JA. Intraperitoneal insulin with CAPD - an artificial pancreas. *Trans Am Soc Artif Intern Organs* 1979, 25:114-117.

MODERN ADVANCES IN PERITONEAL DIALYSIS: AN OVERVIEW

The prevalence of end-stage renal disease continues to increase globally, and most patients are treated with dialysis. Despite technological advances in dialysis care, the relatively high costs of providing dialysis have not decreased substantially over the past 4 decades. The cost benefit of PD is reflected in generally lower expenditure than in-center hemodialysis with the clinical advantages of home therapy. PD offers opportunities of better adequacy, continuous removal of uremic toxins, residual renal function protection, nutritional intraperitoneal support, and life satisfaction. [1, 2].

Each year more than 400 papers are published in the field of peritoneal dialysis highlighting some of the active areas of investigation and development. Advances in controlling peritonitis rates with the Y-set have been dramatic and have resulted in peritonitis rates in many centers less than one episode per 24 patient months. Technique survivals have also improved with lower peritonitis rates. There has been enormous literature on new approaches to treatment and new understandings of host defenses. There are also many advances in peritoneal access. There are now many new types of catheters under investigation such as the Swan-Neck Missouri catheter and the Moncrief-Popovich catheter, with complete burial of the catheter until eventual externalization for CAPD training. There have been major advances in understanding the normal healing of exit sites and the early diagnosis and treatment of exit-site infections.

Trends in Chronic Peritonealdialysis Utilization

Peritoneal dialysis (PD) enjoyed huge growth in the 1980s, followed by a rapid decline in the late 1990s, and a now persistently low utilization rate in many countries, including the United States. Utilization of chronic peritoneal dialysis (CPD) continues to decline in the United States. In 1991, 15% of end-stage renal disease (ESRD) patients were maintained on CPD therapy. That proportion declined to 8.1% in 2002 and to 7% in 2007. This decline is of particular concern because several studies have noted a feeling on the part of nephrologists that more than 30% of ESRD patients should be maintained on CPD therapy [9, 10, 11, 12].

The reported reasons for the decline in utilization have included barriers to the initiation of CPD therapy (problems with education about chronic kidney disease, late referrals, patient preference, and poor social supports, and inadequate structure and function of CPD centers and a proliferation of hemodialysis facilities.

Technique failure (patients switching from one form of dialysis therapy to another) remains a problem for patients maintained on CPD therapy. Technique failure is much higher for CPD patients than for hemodialysis patients [13]. Currently, between 10% and 15% of prevalent CPD patients transfer to hemodialysis each year. The major causes of technique failure include peritonitis, decreased ultrafiltration capacity, problems achieving adequate clearances, and psychosocial issues [13, 14].

Center size has been associated with technique failure. Afolalu et al. noted that technique failure rates are significantly higher in units with fewer than 25 patients than in units with 25 patients or more, and yet mortality rates are similar for those two cohorts [15]. Three other studies examined center size and technique failure rates and suggested that the greater experience in larger units may lead to less technique failure [16, 17, 18].

Efficiency of Peritoneal Dialysis

The efficiency of peritoneal dialysis depends on the volume of fluid infused into the peritoneum at each exchange, the timing of the fluid exchanges and the solute transport properties of the patient's peritoneum. Various techniques have been developed to monitor the function of the peritoneum, which can change with time, particularly if the patient suffers from recurrent peritonitis. The "Quantum" system allows patients to supplement their manual CAPD exchanges with an additional automated exchange during the night. Most APD systems now have programmes that accommodate an extra exchange in the afternoon or evening to supplement the overnight exchanges.

A more radical approach to increasing efficiency has recently been suggested. In "continuous flow" peritoneal dialysis, two catheters or a double lumen catheter are placed in the peritoneal cavity allowing simultaneous infusion and drainage of the fluid [2]. The patient would require dialysis times comparable to overnight APD and the dialysis fluid would have to be produced 'on-line' to make the treatment cost-effective but has the potential to offer solute removal superior to three times weekly hemodialysis [3].

In contrast to hemodialysis, fluid removal from patients receiving peritoneal dialysis is achieved by osmosis. Traditionally, the osmotic agent used in PD fluid has been glucose. Glucose and lactate, the buffer normally used in PD fluid, are both known to be bioincompatible and to have a detrimental effect on peritoneal membrane function [4], limiting the long-term viability of peritoneal dialysis. Prolonged patient exposure to glucose not only influences peritoneal membrane function, but also leads to difficulty in controlling blood glucose in diabetic patients. Glucose absorption can lead to weight gain, which is often coupled with protein malnutrition, in both diabetic and non-diabetic patients. Alternatives to glucose as an osmotic agent have been developed and icodextrin is now commercially available. Icodextrin, a high molecular weight, glucose polymer derived from starch is capable of providing the osmotic force required to sustained fluid removal over prolonged periods (12-16 hour) and has fewer side effects than glucose[5,6].

The ideal buffer to restore the acid-base balance in the body is bicarbonate. In practice, lactate has been used because (unlike bicarbonate) it does not cause precipitation of calcium and magnesium salts in the fluid bags during storage. Modification to the packaging of the fluid, providing a bag with two chambers that can be mixed immediately before use, means that bicarbonate can now be used [7]. Bags with two chambers also allow the glucose to be kept at a low pH when the bag is autoclaved. This dramatically reduces the harmful glucose degradation products present in the solution [8].A third compartment can be added to provide the option of a low or high glucose solution in the same bag. So far, UK renal units have limited experience with these new solutions and the evidence to show that their use preserves peritoneal transport are not yet available.

Preserving Residual Renal Function after Initiation of Dialysis Therapy

Recent clinical data indicate a survival advantage for patients started on PD. Residual renal function is better preserved with PD.

Preserving residual renal function (RRF) after initiation of dialysis therapy is desirable for improving quality of life in ESRD patients. RRF declines more slowly in patients receiving continuous ambulatory peritoneal dialysis (CAPD) than in patients treated with other forms of maintenance dialysis. Episodes of intravascular volume depletion might be expected to cause more rapid loss of RRF, and are more frequent in patients on hemodialysis, which is intermittent therapy [19].

Peritoneal dialysis has been considered as equal renal replacement modality compared to hemodialysis. It is even more advantageous in the protection of the patients' residual renal function, morbidity-mortality indices, and quality of life peritoneal dialysis in the first two years. From economical point of view peritoneal dialysis is less expensive than hemodialysis; therefore in the future its greater role can be expected in the treatment of more and more renal patients. The recently achieved technical development, and also the more widespread use of the automated peritoneal dialysis machines contribute to quality improvement [20, 21].

New peritoneal dialysis (PD) patients have a better survival than new hemodialysis (HD) patients in the first years on dialysis. During long-term treatment, this changes into a survival advantage for HD. The superior initial survival on PD is related to a better preservation of residual renal function of PD patients compared to HD. The importance of residual renal function is probably due to additional properties of native kidneys, such as a better removal of organic acids and low molecular weight proteins than occurs during dialysis. The magnitude of the RRF in PD patients is not only associated with better survival, but also with less uremic symptoms, such as loss of appetite, and also with higher scores on quality of life tests. These relationships are absent for peritoneal clearance. Consequently measures to preserve RRF are extremely important. Studies on an effect of peritoneal transport status on survival have given variable [22].

Peritonitis

Despite technological advances, prevention of peritonitis remains one of the major challenges in peritoneal dialysis (PD). Several innovative developments have shown an impact on peritonitis rates. Innovative antimicrobial-coated catheter modifications have been introduced, showing promising results in vitro. Topical application of antimicrobial agents such as mupirocin to prevent exit-site infections has been successfully used. New alternative agents for topical exit-site care with reduced potential for antimicrobial resistance are under development. Flushing before fill and avoidance of spiking of solution bags has improved peritonitis rates, as have innovative connectology and double-bag systems. Automated PD seems to be superior with regard to peritonitis rates, although clinical evidence for the benefit is not always conclusive. New PD solutions with neutral pH and low concentrations of glucose degradation products (GDPs) have shown beneficial effects on cell viability and have improved peritoneal host defense. Yet despite advantageous clinical outcomes in some studies, other trials with low-GDP solutions did not show any difference in peritonitis rates. The incidence of peritonitis has markedly improved since the end of the 1980s, but the infection remains a significant complication of chronic PD. Quantifying the role of the many practices and devices in reducing complications is difficult, but their combined effect has clearly improved peritonitis outcomes[23].

A large meta-analysis showed that fast transport patients have a 15% increased risk of death, but this is only the case for continuous ambulatory peritoneal dialysis (CAPD) with conventional dialysis solutions. This suggests that the development of over hydration may be the link between transport status and mortality. A fast transport status can be inherent or acquired. The inherent form can either be due to an inflammatory state or to a large mesothelial cell mass. In both situations vasoactive mediators may be locally released. A permanent acquired fast transport status, leading to severe ultrafiltration failure develops in about one third of the patients. It is conceivable that the excess mortality in fast transport patients is caused by the types associated with an inflammatory status and with the acquired type of long-term PD. The latter, linked to morphological peritoneal alterations, is mainly caused by exposure to conventional dialysis solutions. An icodextrin based solution is especially indicated to treat ultrafiltration failure. The aim of the "biocompatible" solutions is to prevent the peritoneal changes. The results of animal and clinical studies are promising so far [22].

In a single-center prospective observational study (2005-2008) of 130 incident urban CAPD patients who started peritoneal dialysis (PD) , 22 first peritonitis episodes was experienced during the 14-month follow-up. Bag exchange evaluation showed that 51.5% of patients washed their hands improperly, 46.2% failed to check expiration date or bag leakage, and 11.5% forgot to wear a face mask and cap. Patients experiencing peritonitis were more likely to forget to wear a face mask and cap. In multivariate Cox regression model, not wearing a face mask and cap [hazard ratio (HR): 7.26; 95% confidence interval (CI): 2.6 to 20.1; $p < 0.001$] and having anemia (HR: 0.96; 95% CI: 0.94 to 0.99; $p = 0.005$) were independent risk factors for a first episode of peritonitis. Not wearing a face mask and cap and having anemia were independent risk factors for peritonitis [24].

References

[1] Klarenbach, S; Manns, B. Economic evaluation of dialysis therapies.Semin Nephrol. 2009, 29(5):524-32.

[2] Rodrigues, A. Cost benefits of peritoneal dialysis in specific groups of patients. Contrib. Nephrol. 2009, 163:285-91.

[3] Gotch FA. Kinetic modeling of continuous flow peritoneal dialysis. Semin Dial. 2001; 14(5):378-83.

[4] Jorres, A; Topley, N; Gahl, GM. Biocompatibility of peritoneal dialysis fluids. Int J Artif Organ. 1992; 15:79-83.

[5] Woodrow, G, Stables, G, Oldroyd, B, Gibson, Turney, JH, Brown john AM. Comparison of icodextrin and glucose solutions for the daytime dwell in automated peritoneal dialysis. Nephrol Dial Transplant 1999; 14:1530-35.

[6] Posthuma, N; ter Wee, PM; Niessen, H; Donker, AJ; Verbrugh, HA; Schalkwijk, CG. Amadori albumin and advanced glycation end-product formation in peritoneal dialysis using icodextrin. Perit Dial Int. 2001; 21:43-51.

[7] Rippe, B; Levin, L. Computer simulations of ultrafiltration profiles for an icodextrin based peritoneal fluid in CAPD. Kidney Int 2000; 57:2546-56.

[8] Gokal, R. Newer peritoneal dialysis solutions. Adv Ren Replace Ther. 2000; 7:302-9.

[9] United States Department of Health and Human Services, Public Health Service, National Institutes of Health, National Institute of Diabetes and

Digestive and Kidney Diseases, U.S. Renal Data System (USRDS). 2009 Annual data report. 2 vols. Bethesda, MD: USRDS; 2009.

[10] Troidle, L; Kliger, AS; Finkelstein, F. Barriers to utilization of chronic peritoneal dialysis in Network #1, New England. Perit Dial Int 2006; 26:452–7.

[11] Mendelssohn, DC; Mullaney, SR; Jung Blake, PG; Mehta, RL. What do American nephrologists think about dialysis modality selection? Am J Kidney Dis 2001; 37:22–9.

[12] Blake, PG; Finkelstein, FO. Why is the proportion of patients doing peritoneal dialysis declining in North America? Perit Dial Int 2001; 21:107–14.

[13] Serkes, KD; Blagg, CR; Nolph, KD; Vonesh, EF; Shapiro. Comparison of patient and technique survival in continuous ambulatory peritoneal dialysis (CAPD) and hemodialysis: a multicenter study. Perit Dial Int 1990; 10:15–19.

[14] Davies, SJ; Phillips, L; Griffiths, AM; Russell, LH; Naish, PF; Russell, I. What really happens to people on long-term peritoneal dialysis? Kidney Int 1998; 54:2207–17.

[15] Afolalu, B; Troidle, L; Osayimwen, O; Bhargava, J, Kitsen; J, Finkelstein, FO. Technique failure and center size in a large cohort of peritoneal dialysis patients in a defined geographic area. Perit Dial Int 2009; 29:292–6.

[16] Huisman, RM; Nieuwenhuizen, MG; Th de Charro F. Patient-related and center-related factors influencing technique survival of peritoneal dialysis in the Netherlands. Nephrol Dial Transplant 2002; 17:1655–60.

[17] Schaubel, DE, Blake, PG, Fenton, SS. Effect of renal center characteristics on mortality and technique failure on peritoneal dialysis. Kidney Int 2001; 60:1517–24.

[18] Guo, A; Mujais, S. Patient and technique survival on peritoneal dialysis in the United States: evaluation in large incident cohorts. Kidney Int Suppl 2003 ;(88):S3–12.

[19] Kuno, T; Matsumoto, K. Clinical benefit of preserving residual renal function in patients after initiation of dialysis. Blood Purif. 2004; 22 Suppl 2:67-71.

[20] Prichard, S. Will peritoneal dialysis be left behind? Semin Dial. 2005, 8(3):167-70.

[21] Krediet, RT. Advances in peritoneal dialysis. Minerva 2007, 9(3):251-60.

[22] Gokal R, Mallick NP. Peritoneal dialysis.*Lancet*. 1999 Mar 6; 353(9155):823-8.

[23] Diaz-Buxo, JA; Himmele, R. Strategies to universally improve peritonitis rates, including use of dialysis solutions with low glucose degradation products. Adv Perit Dial. 2010, 6:37-40.

[24] Dong J, Chen Y.Impact of the bag exchange procedure on risk of peritonitis. Perit Dial Int. 2010 Jul-Aug; 30(4):440-7.

PERITONEAL DIALYSIS: ADVANCES IN TECHNOLOGIES

There have been interesting developments in both technique and technology of peritoneal dialysis in recent years.

Since 1978 when a method of continuous peritoneal dialysis (PD) in the ambulatory patient, PD has been successful as a simple, economical, and effective way to treat stage 5 chronic kidney disease [1]. A number of important innovations in therapy have occurred along the way. The introduction of the "Y-set" catheter connection, incorporating the technology of flushing the tubing lumen before infusing dialysate into the patient after connection, was instrumental in reducing the incidence of PD peritonitis and was a significant advance in the therapy [2, 3].The popularization of nighttime exchanges by an automated cycler system freed the patient from the constraint of having to perform several exchanges during the day. Furthermore, the dosage of dialysis could be adjusted more finely with the cycler, with modifiable variables including dialysate dwell volume, number of exchanges, dwell times, and total overnight treatment times.

Rapid transporters who had problems with fluid removal on conventional continuous ambulatory PD (CAPD) because the longer dwells of CAPD were associated with rapid glucose absorption, dissipation of the osmotic gradient, and poor ultrafiltration could now be more successfully ultrafiltered with the shorter dwell cycles on the automated PD.

Technologic advances rarely result in immediate improvement in clinical outcome; they require rigorous study and sufficient observation time. The low incidence of peritonitis in recent years and the general use of modern disconnect systems, proving the beneficial effect of any connector on peritonitis incidence is difficult.

REFERENCES

[1] Popovich, R; Moncrief, J; Nolph, K.Continuous ambulatory peritoneal dialysis. *Artif Organs 1978,* 2: 84–86.

[2] Maiorca, R; Cantaluppi, A; Canacarini, G; et al. Prospective controlled trial of a Y-connector and disinfectant to prevent peritonitis in continuous ambulatory peritoneal dialysis. *Lancet* 1983, 2: 642–644,

[3] Canadian CAPD Clinical Trials Group: Peritonitis in continuous ambulatory peritoneal dialysis (CAPD): A multicentre randomized clinical trial comparing the Y connector disinfectant system to standard systems. *Perit Dial Int* 1989, 9: 159–163.

NEW BIOCOMPATIBLE PERITONEAL DIALYSIS SOLUTIONS

PD solutions play an increasingly important role in current peritoneal dialysis research and development. In the 1920s, Ganter used a physiological saline solution, to which glucose was added later. In 1938, Jonathan Rhoads began adding lactate to the solution to correct metabolic acidosis, which can develop if the kidneys are unable to eliminate acidic metabolic products. More than 60 years later, lactate remains the most commonly used buffer in PD solution.

In 1981, Axel Duwe and his colleagues published an article about the effects of individual components of PD solution on peritoneal efficiency on bacterial killing for the first time [1]. They reported that commercial fluids used in peritoneal dialysis suppress the activity of peripheral blood leukocytes as measured by chemiluminescence, phagocytosis, and bacterial killing. Suppression was found to be due to the low pH and high osmolality of the fluid. They adjusted pH to non-inhibitory levels in vivo within 30 min, whereas osmolality changes were less rapid and remained at inhibitory levels for fluids of high dextrose concentration (4.25%). Chemiluminescence's was the most sensitive assay for inhibitory effects of pH and osmolality, as well as for urea and heparin. The metabolic waste product urea at levels normally found in dialysate and heparin at concentrations routinely added to fluid inhibited only chemiluminescence, whereas creatinine and added insulin were not inhibitory. High fluid volume also resulted in a decrease in efficiency of bacterial killing. Axel and his colleagues suggested some changes to be made in peritoneal dialysis.

A few years later the term “bio (in) compatibility” appeared to indicate the body’s (in) tolerance of dialysis solutions. At the time, studies showed that conventional PD solutions could inhibit the activities of key cells in the peritoneum and cause long-term damage to the membrane. These complications led to a gradual weakening of the peritoneal membrane and make it unsuitable for further use as a dialyzer. Conventional dialysis solutions have a non-physiological pH below that of the peritoneum and a high concentration of glucose degradation products. Both contribute significantly to the bioincompatibility of solutions [2-7]. Now, PD solutions are offered in multi-chamber bags that have a neutral to physiological pH and a significantly lower amount of glucose degradation products. There are also solutions containing pure bicarbonate or a mixture of the two substances, bicarbonate and lactate, to balance the acid-base status. As a substitute for glucose, dialysis solutions can also contain amino acids or glucose polymers.

Long-term peritoneal dialysis (PD) can lead to morphologic and functional alterations of the peritoneum [2]. These alterations are probably caused by chronic exposure to bioincompatible dialysis solutions. Extremely high concentrations of glucose and the presence of glucose degradation products are among the most important culprits [3].

Conventional peritoneal dialysis (PD) fluids are acidic and contain high levels of glucose degradation products (GDPs) as a result of the heat sterilization process. During sterilization and extended storage periods, dextrose degrades into GDPs, which are potentially harmful molecules. The dextrose molecule naturally interconverts between an annular and a linear structure. In aqueous solution, the linear dextrose molecule exists in equilibrium with 1, 2-enediol, which is susceptible to degradation reactions.

Under elevated temperatures and in mildly acidic conditions (the pH range typical of conventional PD solutions), 1, 2-enediol will form 3-deoxyaldose-2-ene, which in turn forms the GDPs 3-deoxyglucosone (3-DG) and 3, 4-dideoxyglucosone-3-ene (3, 4-DGE). The 3, 4-DGE will then decompose into 5-hydroxymethyfurfural (5-HMF). The GDPs, glyoxal (Glx), methylglyoxal (M-Glx), and furaldehyde stem from 1, 2-enediol and 3-deoxyaldose-2-ene decomposition. Dextrose also react with lactate (present in most PD fluids as an osmotic agent and pH buffer) to form acetaldehyde (AcA) during heat sterilization [4, 5, 6, 7].

Standard peritoneal solutions must be stable with a practicable shelf life. Because the solution is very high in glucose, a major byproduct of this solution is the formation of glucose degradation products (GDP). These comprise a family of compounds with known or suspected adverse consequences, both at the level of the peritoneal membrane and also systemically, via absorption from the peritoneal cavity [8]. The GDP can also link with proteins, leading to the formation of advanced glycosylation end products. An ambient acidic pH will reduce the formation of GDP in the bag of dialysate, and for this reason, the pH of unused peritoneal dialysate is approximately 5.2.

Another challenge with formulating peritoneal dialysate for storage is that bicarbonate cannot be used as the buffer, because it has the potential to react with calcium in the dialysate and form calcium-carbonate precipitates. Therefore, lactate is used in lieu of bicarbonate and is rapidly and successfully converted into bicarbonate *in* vivo. Given the acid pH (but not sufficiently acidic to halt completely the formation of GDP), high lactate, and absent bicarbonate, peritoneal dialysate is not completely physiologic, or "biocompatible." A number of studies using both in vivo and in vitro methods have suggested that the standard dialysate is associated with depletion of mesothelial cells that line the peritoneal cavity, thickening of the membrane itself, and the development of a unique vasculopathy of the vessels in the peritoneal interface [9,10,11].It has been postulated that nonphysiologic components of the dialysate, in inducing these anatomic changes, may ultimately lead to the development of rapid-transport status and ultrafiltration failure that is seen in a subset of long-term PD patients. This observation has prompted the ingenious development of PD solutions that have been labeled as "biocompatible." The dialysate is divided into at least two subcompartments. One compartment contains the glucose and the electrolytes. This subcompartment has a very low pH, which slows the formation of GDP. The other compartment contains bicarbonate or a bicarbonate-lactate mixture. Because the calcium is stored in the glucose-containing compartment, separated from the buffer, there is no risk for calcium-bicarbonate interaction during storage.

Before the dialysis exchange, the patient breaks a frangible connection that separates the two compartments, and when the components are mixed, the final pH is close to physiologic. The patient now infuses a normal-pH, low-GDP, bicarbonate-containing solution [12, 13].

A major, well-conducted, randomized, controlled, crossover trial found, in a secondary end point, that urine volume and residual renal GFR increased when the patient was using the biocompatible dialysis fluid and decreased with the standard dialysate [14].Indeed, in this crossover format, the patients who started with the standard solution had an increase in urine volume when crossed over to the biocompatible dialysis fluid. These results were interpreted as showing that the biocompatible fluid "preserved" residual renal function. What is not appreciated in this study, however, is that there was a change in the peritoneal transport characteristics associated with the new solutions. Indeed, the so-called biocompatible solution was associated with a change to a more rapid transporter phenotype, with consequent reduction in ultrafiltration of 350 ml/d. (It is relevant to remember that one explanation for the higher incidence of congestive heart failure in the control group in the Adequacy of Peritoneal Dialysis in Mexico [ADEMEX] trial was a reduction in ultrafiltration of approximately 100 ml/d.) The contribution of this reduced ultrafiltration and change in volume status to the increase in residual renal function is unclear.

Two recent reports from Korea examined survival in PD patients who underwent dialysis with conventional versus newer neutral-pH solutions. Theses non-randomized studies found that patients who underwent dialysis with the biocompatible dialysate lived longer compared with those who did not [15, 16]. There were differences in center characteristics between the two groups, and the younger age of the group that received the biocompatible dialysate alone accounted for half of the mortality difference.

In addition, a very long-living subset of patients who started therapy on standard solutions and were switched to the newer solutions were correctly included as part of the standard group in the intention-to-treat analysis in the first publication [15] but removed from the analysis altogether in the second report [16]. This can lead to a major problem of confounding by indication, in that the physicians may decide to "invest" in the healthier patients and switch them over to the newer, expensive PD solutions.

Although these solutions could lead to less damage by GDP and a small relative reduction in circulating levels of advanced glycosylation end products, extrapolating this to preservation of residual renal function and prolongation of life still remains a big leap. Early findings of reduction in peritonitis have not been reproduced [15, 16].

One study showed that, compared with a conventional dialysis solution, a mixture of osmotic agents and bicarbonate/lactate buffer [glycerol 1.4%, amino acids 0.5%, dextrose 1.1% (GLAD)] used in a peritoneal exposure model in rats with renal failure resulted in a reduced number of peritoneal vessels[17]. However, transport of small solutes was not reduced. We hypothesized that these unexpected findings might be attributable to vasodilation. Dilation of peritoneal vessels can be caused by exposure to amino acids or by upregulation of endothelial NO synthase (eNOS). A study in stable PD patients exposed to an amino acid–based solution (as compared with a glucose-based solution) showed higher peritoneal blood flow and higher mass transfer area coefficients (MTACs) of small solutes. This effect was independent of vasodilating prostaglandins, and it was also unlikely to be mediated by NO [18]. On the other hand, uremic rats have showed increased expression of eNOS and a beneficial effect of NOS inhibition by *N*γ -nitro-L-arginine methyl ester (L-NAME) on permeability changes during peritonitis[19,20].Production of NO can be inhibited by L-arginine analogs [21] such as L-NAME and *N*γ -monomethyl-Larginine (L-NMMA). The latter is able to inhibit both constitutive and inducible NO synthase [22].

One of the main goals in the development of dialysis techniques is to use materials and chemicals, in concentration and composition as close as possible to those found in the body. Lactate is practically the only dialysate buffer currently used in PD; there are still many doubts about the metabolic tolerance of chronic exposure to high concentrations of this molecule. Lactate represents the end product of glucose catabolism in the Embden-Meyerhof pathway (EMP), which accounts for approximately 90% of total glucose metabolism in the resting cell [23, 24, 25]. In the red cell, this pathway produces energy, which is then stored in the high energy phosphate of ATP, and the reducing power used in the conversion of NAD+ to NADH. This coenzyme participates in the transformation of methemoglobin to hemoglobin. Lactate containing buffers may have a metabolic impact on the cell where, before the conversion to bicarbonate which takes place in liver and muscle cells, it accumulates. Furthermore, its infusion takes place at a pH of about 5.5-5.7.

The mechanism of pH buffering by lactate administration is based on pure compensatory respiratory acidosis, which results from the stimulation of the central nervous system by massive lactate infusion [26]. A late and long-lasting metabolic compensation of pH is then obtained with a net gain in the bicarbonate concentration; conversion of lactate to bicarbonate is mainly due to the hepatic and muscular metabolism [27]. Since bicarbonate is the physiological buffer in the blood, bicarbonate infusion allows a direct compensation of the cellular pH. The intracellular H+ accumulation is prevented by bicarbonate consumption through the carbonic anhydrase reaction; the CO2produced is then eliminated through an appropriate ventilatory response. Under acidotic conditions, bicarbonate consumption then occurs as a consequence of the CO2 elimination and this is the reason why the dialysate should be supplemented with a buffer (bicarbonate or any other buffer) able to re store it.

Available evidence suggests a deleterious effect of lactate buffer in the RBC of PD Patients, who is not observed when bicarbonate buffer is used. The damaging effect of lactate on RBC metabolism causes energy depletion (low energy charge levels). While this aspect correlates in vitra with an acute inhibition of some key enzymes in the EMP, in PD patients a compensatory activation of glycolysis (increased activity of the key enzyme in this pathway) can be hypothesized as a result of the in viva action of lactate. Our results also demonstrate that G-3-PD activity is one of the most probable targets of the action of lactate on the glycolytic pathway. Both our in viva and in vitra experiments demonstrated that red cell pH is physiologically and readily restored by the bicarbonate based solutions, while the lactate based counterparts with acidic composition induce a condition of acidosis in the cellular compartment, which may persist if inadequate conditions for the lactate metabolization are present. Lactate infusion induces cell damage by a multi-factorial mechanism including the direct metabolic effect of its accumulation, its oxidative properties and pH lowering. Thus, the replacement of lactate with bicarbonate in PD solutions eliminates these drawbacks and is theoretically advantageous for the metabolism and function of cells, including those not in direct contact with the solution [28].

Recently, a dialysis solution containing icodextrin as the osmotic agent has been widely used in peritoneal dialysis. Icodextrin-based peritoneal dialysis solution (icodextrin) contains a polyglucose prepared by hydrolysis of starch. The mean molecular weight (MW) of icodextrin is as large as 16,800 Da, and differences in colloid osmotic pressure induce water transport.I codextrin is absorbed slowly into the blood causing persistent osmotic pressure differences contributing to sufficient ultrafiltration in patients with increased peritoneal membrane permeability . However, the development of allergic dermatologic responses such as erythema, bulla, and exfoliative dermatitis have been reported in 2.5% – 15% of PD patients who use icodextrin [29, 30, 31]. Severe cases of allergic dermatitis [32] and sterile peritonitis [33] have also been reported in association with the use of icodextrin-based solutions. Therefore, the biocompatibility and effects of icodextrin on the peritoneum have become matters of concern.

It is still too early to know whether the new solutions will delay the development of late ultrafiltration failure in long-term PD patients. A rapid-transport state is associated with inflammation and vasodilation of vascular beds in the peritoneum, the increase, rather than decrease, in transperitoneal solute flux with these new solutions remains a concern. However, there is still a sound physiologic underpinning to the design of the newer solutions. What is needed, however, are rigorous controlled trials to prove that biocompatibility translates into better patient outcomes.

References

[1] Duwe, AK; S I Vas, SI; Weatherhead, JW. Effects of the composition of peritoneal dialysis fluid on chemiluminescence, phagocytosis, and bactericidal activity in vitro. *Infect Immun* 1981; 33(1): 130–135.

[2] De Vriese, AS; Mortier, S; Lameire NH. What happens to the peritoneal membrane in long-term peritoneal dialysis? *Perit Dial Int* 2001, 21(Suppl 3):S9–18.

[3] Davies, SJ; Phillips, L; Naish, PF; Russell, I. Peritoneal glucose exposure and changes in membrane solute transport with time on peritoneal dialysis. J Am Soc Nephrol 2001, 12:1046–51.

[4] Anet, E. Degradation of carbohydrates. *Austr J Chem* 1962, 15:503–9.

[5] Anet, E. 3-Deoxyglycosuloses (3-deoxyglycosones) and the degradation of carbohydrates. Adv Carbohydr Chem 1964, 19:181–218.

[6] Linden, T; Cohen, A; Deppisch, R; Kjellstrand, P; Wieslander, A. 3, 4-Dideoxyglucosone-3-ene (3, 4-DGE): a cytotoxic glucose degradation product in fluids for peritoneal dialysis. *Kidney Int* 2002, 62:697–703.

[7] Wieslander, AP; Deppisch, R; Svensson, E; et alvitro biocompatibility of a heat sterilized, low-toxic, and less acidic fluid for peritoneal dialysis. *Perit Dial Int* 1995, 5:158–64.

[8] Zeier, M; Schwenger, V; Deppisch, R; et al. Glucose degradation products in PD fluids: Do they disappear from the peritoneal cavity and enter the systemic circulation? *Kidney Int* 2003, 63: 298–305.

[9] Combet, S; Miyata, T; Moulin, P; et al. Vascular proliferation and enhanced expression of endothelial nitric oxide synthase in human peritoneum exposed to long-term peritoneal dialysis. *J Am Soc Nephrol* 2000, 11: 717–728.

[10] Yanez-Mo, M; Lara-Pezzi, E; Selgas, R; et al. Peritoneal dialysis and epithelial-to-mesenchymal transition of mesothelial cells. *N Engl J Med* 2003, 348: 403–413.

[11] Wong; Phillips, A; Witowski, J; Topley N.Glucose-mediatedinduction of TGF-beta 1 and MCP-1 in mesothelial cells in vitro is osmolality and polyol pathway dependent. *Kidney Int* 2003, *63*: 1404–1416.

[12] Simonsen, O; Wieslander, A; Landgren, C; Rippe, B. Less infusion pain and elevated level of cancer antigen 125 by the use of a new and more biocompatible PD fluid. *Adv Perit Dial* 1996, *12*: 156–160.

[13] Feriani, M; Kirchgessner, J; La Greca, G; Passlick-Deetjen, J.Bicarbonate CAPD Cooperative Group: Randomized long-term evaluation of bicarbonate-buffered CAPD solution. *Kidney Int* 1998, 54: 1731–1738.

[14] Williams, J; Topley N; Craig, K; Mackenzie ,R;et al.The Euro-Balance Trial: The effect of a new biocompatible peritoneal dialysis fluid (balance) on the peritoneal membrane. *Kidney Int* 2004, 66: 408–418.

[15] Lee, H; Park, H; Seo, B; Do J; et al. Superior patient survival for continuous ambulatory peritoneal dialysis patients treated with a peritoneal dialysis fluid with neutral pH and low glucose degradation product concentration (balance). *Perit Dial Int* 2005, 25: 248–255.

[16] Lee, H; Choi, H; Park, H; et al. Changing prescribing practice in CAPD patients in Korea: Increased utilization of low GDP solutions improves patient outcome. *Nephrol Dial Transplant* 2006, 21: 2893–2899.

[17] de Graaff, M; Zegwaard, AH; Zweers, MM; et al. The effects of a dialysis solution with a combination of glycerol/amino acids/dextrose on the peritoneal membrane in chronic renal failure. Perit Dial Int 2010, 30:192–200.

[18] Douma, CE; de Waart, DR; Struijk, DG; Krediet, RT. Effect of amino acid based dialysate on peritoneal blood flow and permeability in stable CAPD patients: a potential role for nitric oxide? Clin Nephrol 1996, 45:295–302.

[19] Combet, S; Ferrier, ML; Landschoot van, M; et al. Chronic uremia induces permeability changes, increased nitric oxide synthase expression, and structural modifications in the peritoneum. J Am Soc Nephrol 2001, 12:2146–57.

[20] Ferrier, ML; Combet, S; Landschoot van M; et al. Inhibition of nitric oxide synthase reverses changes in peritoneal permeability in a rat model of acute peritonitis. Kidney Int 2001, 60:2343–50.

[21] Gross, SS; Stuehr, DJ; Aisaka, K; et al. Macrophage and endothelial cell nitric oxide synthesis: cell-type selective inhibition by NGaminoarginine, NG-nitroarginine and NGmethylarginine. Biochem Biophys Res Commun 1990, 170:96–103.

[22] Lambert, LE; Whitten, JP; Baron, BM; et al. Nitric oxide synthesis in the CNS endothelium and macrophages differs in its sensitivity to inhibition by arginine analogues. Life Sci 1991, 48:69–75.

[23] Zhou,XJ;Yu,AW;Zhou,FQ;et al. Neutrophil intracellular pH after exposure of neutrophils to a euhydric, lactate-based peritoneal dialysis solution and its euhydric, bicarbonate-based counterpart. *Int J Artif Organs* 1995; 18 69-72.

[24] Ing, TS; Wong, FKM; YangML; et al. Acidic, DL-pyruvate-based peritoneal dialysis solutions: relationship between low titratable acidity and biocompatibility. *Perit Dial Int* 1995; 15(Suppl):S33.

[25] Ing, TS; Wong, FKM; Yu, AW; et al. Effect of an acidic, DL-pyruvate-based or an acidic, DL-Iactate-based peritoneal dialysis solution (PDS) on neutrophilic oxygen consumption. *Perit Dial Int* 1995; 15(Suppl):S33.

[26] Panichi, V; Parrini, M; Bianchi, AM*; et al.* Mechanisms of acid base homeostasis in acetate and bicarbonate dialysis, lactate hemofiltration and hemodiafiltration. *Int J Artif Organs* 1994; 12:315-21.

[27] Gollnick PD, Hermansen L, Yunis JJ. Biochemical adaptations to exercise: anaerobic metabolism. In: Exercise and sport sciences reviews. New York: Academic Press; 1973; 1:1-39.

[28] Buoncristiani, U; Galli, F; Rovidati, S; et al. Bicarbonate versus lactate buffer in peritoneal dialysis solutions: the beneficial effect on RBC metabolism. *Perit Dial Int* 1996; 16: 511-518.

[29] Wolfson, M; Piraino, B; Hamburger, RJ; Morton, AR, for the Icodextrin Study Group. A randomized controlled trial to evaluate the efficacy and safety of icodextrin in peritoneal dialysis. *Am J Kidney Dis* 2002; 40:1055–65.

[30] Goldsmith, D; Jayawardene, S; Sabharwal, N; Cooney K. Allergic reactions to the polymeric glucose-based peritoneal dialysis fluid icodextrin in patients with renal failure. *Lancet* 2000; 355:897.

[31] Divino Fiho, JC. Allergic reactions to icodextrin in patients with renal failure. *Lancet* 2000; 355:1364–5.

[32] Queffeulou, G; Bernard, M; Vrtovsnik, F; *et al.* Severe cutaneous hypersensitivity requiring permanent icodextrin withdrawal in a CAPD patient. *Clin Nephrol* 1999; 51:184–6.

[33] Toure, F; Lavaud, S; Mohajer, M; *et al.* Icodextrin induced peritonitis: study of five cases and comparison with bacterial peritonitis. *Kidney Int* 2004; 65: 654–60.

NEW PD CATHETER PLACEMENT TECHNIQUES

A nonfunctioning or poorly functioning PD catheter is a major cause of technique failure and a hindrance to the establishment of a successful PD program. Whereas hemodialysis has the tunneled or non-tunneled internal jugular line as a default option for the patient who is unable to maintain a fistula or a graft, there is no equivalent for the PD patient, who will then be forced to change dialysis modality.

Research has proposed various valid solutions to solve the problem of peritoneal access during peritoneal dialysis (PD) [1–5]. Since the first application of this technique in 1923 [2], many catheters of different forms have been tried, until the creation of the Maxwell semi-rigid catheter [3], which enabled the first true development of acute PD. The possibility of chronic PD came about with the invention of the Tenckhoff catheter [4], which is still valid and widely used today. Indeed, all new catheters proposed and used since then have been slight modifications of the Tenckhoff catheter.

In the past 20 years, various modifications in form, composition, and insertion technique have been proposed [5]. The ideal peritoneal catheter [6] must provide an effective barrier to infectious agents between the peritoneal cavity and the outside; it must have good biocompatibility; it must not become displaced; it must not leak; it must enable simple, repeatable long-term access to the peritoneum.

Over the years, new forms and materials, and biocompatibility, have been studied to eliminate or reduce the main complications, namely, infection of the subcutaneous tunnel and exit site, dislocation of the catheter, peritonitis, and general malfunctioning of the catheter [1, 4, 5]. One of the main disadvantages of the Tenckhoff catheter is dislocation of the catheter tip [7]. Dislocation may be small, with the tip remaining in the lowermost part of the abdominal cavity, or large, with the tip migrating into the upper abdomen [8]. Dislocation is often accompanied by obstruction of the holes in the catheter by omentum, which is absent in the Douglas cavity. It may impair dialysis [7, 9–11], causing slow and/or inadequate outflow, leakage, pain on filling, inefficient dialysis, or cessation of outflow [12].

Some evidence shows that the use of catheters with a permanent bend in the intramural segment is beneficial, because these catheters are associated with fewer episodes of early outflow obstruction and catheter migration as compared with straight catheters traversing an arcuate tunnel, and these may be associated with a reduced incidence of catheter infection. Use of swan-neck catheters is increasing [13-17]. In the 1994 [13], a dramatic increase in their use was noted in North America, and it now seems that Europe is following the same trend. A committee of the International Society for Peritoneal Dialysis [15, 16] suggested that preferential use of catheters with permanent bend might be beneficial. Double-cuff catheters continue to be preferred over single-cuff catheters by both adult and pediatric centers. The intraperitoneal segment of PD catheters can be coiled or straight. The coiled catheter is associated with less inflow pain, and was preferentially used in the adult. In a recent systematic review of available randomized controlled trials of peritoneal catheters, straight and coiled intraperitoneal segments were found to be associated with similar rates of peritonitis, exit-site and tunnel infection, and catheter removal and replacement events [18].

Options for placement techniques include conventional surgical insertion, insertion under peritoneoscopic or laparoscopic guidance, "blind" insertion, and radiologic insertion with fluoroscopy. It has been considered that the particular method of insertion is not as important for the success of the catheter as much as the experience and the interest of the operator performing the insertion. Because the nephrologist has an interest in the success of the catheter, it is not surprising that good results have been reported with the techniques when the nephrologists perform the procedure [19]. However, many nephrologists do not have the time, training, or inclination to insert peritoneal catheters. In that case, the insertion usually falls to a surgeon. Again, results may be predicated on the interest or the experience of the surgeon. In addition, blind surgical placement can be hampered by stool-filled bowel, a lively omentum, and bowel adhesions.

Laparoscopic PD catheter insertion

Insertion of the dialysis catheter under direct visualization by laparoscopy affords a number of advantages. The operator can ensure, in real time, that the catheter tip is placed in the deep pelvis. Adhesions can be lysed during the procedure, and a large, redundant omentum can be tacked up into the upper abdomen ("omentopexy") to prevent it from wrapping around the catheter tip in the pelvis. Furthermore, the part of the catheter that traverses the rectus sheath in the abdominal wall can be tunneled superinferiorly so that the catheter has a "built in" directionality into the pelvis and decreases the chances of its flipping into the middle or upper abdomen.

Excellent results have been reported with the insertion techniques using direct visualization. Crabtree et al. [20] noted very high rates of primary and long-term function with laparoscopic placement of peritoneal catheters, compared with their experience with the blind surgical technique. Conversely, others have had very good experience with blind placement or placement with the aid of a peritoneoscope (where placement and visualization can be done only in sequence, not simultaneously).

The literature has been contradictory in terms of comparisons between laparoscopic and surgical insertions [21, 22]. A recent review and meta-analysis of randomized trials that compared laparoscopy with laparotomy reported no significant difference in peritonitis, catheter replacement, or technique failure [23]. In the final analysis, the most important predictor of successful catheter implantation is likely having an operator who is committed to and engaged in the procedure.

Nonetheless, the laparoscopic technique affords the surgeon a greater degree of visualization and control over the proper placement of the catheter and the opportunity to deal with impediments such as intraperitoneal adhesions.

Buried PD Catheters

Another relatively new technique is the method of "burying" the distal end of the newly implanted PD catheter subcutaneously so that no part of the catheter is extracutaneous. The original intent of this technique, proposed by Moncrief et al. [24], to allow complete healing of the catheter tunnel in a sterile environment. By avoiding unintended bacterial inoculation of the catheter, exit site, or tunnel, a germ-free seal could be formed during the wound healing. After a period of time, originally proposed as 3 to 5 wk, the distal end of the catheter could be externalized.

A recent analysis of randomized studies that compared this technique with standard implantation showed no difference in exit-site or tunnel infection rate (two trials, 2511 patient months; relative risk 0.90; 95% confidence interval 0.39 to 2.08) or a significant reduction in peritonitis (relative risk 1.16; 95% confidence interval 0.37 to 3.60) [25]. Although results have perhaps been disappointing with regard to prevention of catheter-associated infections, the Moncrief technique has been revisited as a method to implant a PD catheter preemptively. Because the whole catheter is subcutaneous or deeper, there is no risk for exit-site infection or inoculation at the time of implantation and no need (and indeed no access) for flushing of the catheter. In theory, the catheter could stay unused for months or even years and then quickly mobilized by an externalization procedure that can be done in the office or the bedside and used immediately for PD. In this way, the buried catheter could be, similar to early construction of an arteriovenous fistula for hemodialysis, part of good predialysis planning for patients, enabling them to have ideal access in place at the time of commencement of dialysis, even when dialysis has to be started urgently.

Because the catheter is to be inserted and left without access to flushing, it is crucial that the implantation technique proceed so that the intraluminal portion does not fill with clot or with fibrin and that the omentum is not activated and wraps around the intraperitoneal portion of the catheter. There have been previous reports of these complications with the embedded technique [26]. However, with careful attention to these issues during the implantation, the buried technique can be a useful way to secure peritoneal access ahead of time so that the patient can start either electively or urgently with this modality, rather than risking interim insertion of a temporary hemodialysis catheter [27].

Self-locating catheter

A self-locating catheter has been constructed. The catheter retains the classic Tenckhoff form, except in the final 2 cm, where the external diameter is slightly larger and the usual perforations are absent. Internal diameter is the same as in the original, and the distance between he internal cuff and the tip is 16 cm instead f the original 15 cm. Twelve grams of tungsten, a physically and chemically inert element, are sufficient or continuous self-positioning of the tip in the lowest point of the Douglas cavity, without altering catheter function, causing discomfort, or interfering with the organs it contacts. It can be inserted by the methods used for the Tenckhoff catheter or by a keyhole technique involving the use of a specially designed steel insertion forceps, an insertion needle (16 gauge × 7 cm), a flexible steel guide (50 cm ×1 mm), a rigid round-ended mandrel, and an echotomographic guide (28,29,30).

A multicenter control study confirmed demonstrated that complications of peritoneal dialysis, such as cuff extrusion, infection, peritonitis, early leakage, and obstruction, are statistically less frequent in patients with self-locating catheters than in patients with classic Tenckhoff catheters[31].

REFERENCES

[1] Piraino, B. Which catheter is the best buy? *Perit Dial Int* 1995; 15:303–4.

[2] Ganter, G. Uber die Beseitingung giftiger Stoffe aus dem Blute durch Dialyse. *Munch Med Wochenschr* 1923; 70:1478–80.

[3] Maxwell, MH; Rockney, RE; Kleeman, CR; Twiss, MR. Peritoneal dialysis. *JAMA* 1959; 170:917.

[4] Tenckhoff, H; Schechter, H. A bacteriologically safe peritoneal access device. *Trans Am Soc Artif Intern Organs* 1968; 14:181.

[5] Nielsen, P; Hemmingsen, C; Ladefoged, J; Olgaard, K. A consecutive study of 646 peritoneal dialysis catheters. *Perit Dial Int* 1994; 14:170–2.

[6] Oreopoulos, DG; Izatt, S; Zellerman, G. A prospective study of the effectiveness of three permanent peritoneal catheters. *Proc Clin Dial Transplant Forum* 1976; 6:96–100.

[7] Vogt, K; Binswanger, U; Buchman, P. Catheter-related complications during CAPD: a retrospective study on sixty-two double-cuff Tenckhoff catheters. *Am J Kidney Dis* 1987; 10:47–51.

[8] Di Paolo, N; Petrini, G; Garosi, G; et al. A new self-locating peritoneal catheter. *Perit Dial Int* 1996; 16:623–7.

[9] Biermann, MH; Kasperbauer, J; Kusek, A; et al. Peritoneal catheter survival and complications in end-stage renal disease. *Perit Dial Bull* 1985; 5:229–33.

[10] Twardowski, ZJ. Malposition and poor drainage of peritoneal catheters. *Semin Dial* 1990; 3:57.

[11] Julian, TB; Ribeiro, U; Bruns, F. Malfunctioning peritoneal dialysis catheter repaired by laparoscopic surgery. *Perit Dial Int* 1995; 15:363–6.

[12] Shyr, YM. Complications of peritoneal catheters placed by a single surgeon. *Perit Dial Int* 1994; 14:401–3.

[13] Twardowski, ZJ; Nolph, KD; Khanna, R; Prowant, BF. Computer interaction: catheters. *Adv Perit Dial* 1994; 10:11–18.

[14] Twardowski, ZJ. History of peritoneal access development *Int J Artif Organs* 2006; 29:2–40.

[15] Gokal, R; Alexander, S; Ash, S; *et al.* Peritoneal catheters and exit-site practices toward optimum peritoneal access: 1998 update. Official Report from the International Society for Peritoneal Dialysis. *Perit Dial Int* 1998; 18:11–33.

[16] Flanigan M, Gokal R. Peritoneal catheters and exit site practices toward optimum peritoneal access: a review of current developments. Perit Dial Int 2005; 25:132–9.

[17] Thodis, E; Passadakis, P; Lyrantzopooulos, N; et al. Peritoneal catheters and related infections. *Int Urol Nephrol* 2005; 37:379–93.

[18] Strippoli, GF; Tong, A; Johnson, D; Schena, FP; Craig, JC. Catheter-related interventions to prevent peritonitis in peritoneal dialysis: a systematic review of randomized, controlled trials. *J Am Soc Nephrol* 2004; 15:2735-46.

[19] Asif, A; Pflederer, T; Viera, C; Diego J; et al. Does catheter insertion by nephrologists improve peritoneal dialysis utilization? A multicenter analysis. *Semin Dial* 2005, 18: 157–160,

[20] Crabtree, J, Fishman, A.A laparoscopic method for optimal peritoneal dialysis access. *Am Surg* 2005, 71: 135–143.

[21] Soontrapornchai, P; Simapatanapong, T.Comparison of open and laparoscopic secure placement of peritoneal dialysis catheters. *Surg Endosc* 2005, 19: 137–139.

[22] Lu, C; Watson, D; Elias, T; et al. Laparoscopic placement of peritoneal dialysis catheters: 7 years experience. *ANZ J Surg* 2003, 73: 109–111.

[23] Strippoli, G; Tong, A; Johnson, D; Schena F; Craig J. Catheter- related interventions to prevent peritonitis in peritoneal dialysis: A systematic review of randomized, controlled trials. *J Am Soc Nephrol* 2004,15: 2735–2746.

[24] Moncrief, J; Popovich, R; Broadrick, L; et al.The Moncrief-Popovich catheter. A new peritoneal access technique for patients on peritoneal dialysis. *ASAIO J* 1993, 39: 62–65.

[25] Strippoli G, Tong A, Johnson D, Schena F, Craig J: Catheter-related interventions to prevent peritonitis in peritoneal dialysis: A systematic review of randomized, controlled trials. *J Am Soc Nephrol* 2004, 15: 2735–2746.

[26] Prischl, F; Wallner, M; Kalchmair, H; et al. Initial subcutaneous embedding of the peritoneal dialysis catheter: A critical appraisal of this new implantation technique. *Nephrol Dial Transplant* 12: 1661–1667, 1997

[27] McCormick, B; Brown, P; Knoll, G; et al. Use of the embedded peritoneal dialysis catheter: Experience and results from a North American Center. *Kidney Int Suppl* 2006, 103: S38–S43.

[28] Cavagna, R; Tessarin, C; Tarroni, G; et al. The self-locating catheter: clinical evaluation and comparison with the Tenckhoff catheter. *Perit Dial Int* 1999; 19:540–3.
[29] Minguela,I; Lanuza,M; Ruiz De Guana,R; Rodado,R; Aòlegria,S. Lower malfunction rate with self-locating catheters. *Perit Dial Int* 2001; 21(Suppl 3):S209–12.
[30] Di Paolo, N; Manganelli, A; Strappaveccia, F; De Mia, M; Gaggiotti, E. A new technique for insertion of Tenckhoff peritoneal dialysis catheter. *Nephron* 1985; 40: 485–7.
[31] Paolo, ND; Capotondo, L; Sansoni, E; et al. The self-locating catheter: clinical experience and follow-up. *Perit Dial Int2004;* 24: 359–364.

ADVANCES IN BAG CONNECTION TECHNOLOGY

Several modifications of the continuous ambulatory peritoneal dialysis (CAPD) technique over the last decades were introduced, including advances in bag connection technology [1, 2].

There are three main types of delivery (catheter connecting) systems in use today.

The simple spike (straight connecting system) was considered as the 'standard' system during the 1980s. In this system, the catheter is connected to the bag via a piece of tubing and a spike or a Luer lock device. During each bag exchange procedure, the spent dialysate is drained from the peritoneal cavity into the empty bag, which is then disconnected and discarded. A new bag is then connected to the patient's permanent catheter and the fresh dialysate is introduced into the peritoneal cavity. The empty bag is rolled up and remains attached to the patient until the next bag exchange (non-disconnecting system).

The second delivery system is the Y-set (Y-System with empty bag) in which the patient disconnects from the bags between exchanges (disconnect system). Umberto Buoncristiani from Italy was the first to describe the Y-System. This system includes an empty bag and connected tubes shaped like a "Y" dictating the flow of dialysis solution. A bag filled with PD solution is connected to this system. First of all, the used dialysis solution is drained into the empty bag, carrying possible bacteria from the catheter connector. Then fresh dialysis solution is flushed through the tubes and into the bag for about three seconds. The connection to the abdominal cavity remains closed during this procedure. When the tubes have been flushed, the patient's catheter connector is opened and fresh PD solution is introduced into the cavity (flush-before-fill principle). Depending on the system, the flow of PD solution (drainage, flush, filling) is controlled with clamps or a disc. This technology plays an essential part in lowering the peritonitis rate. Any microorganisms that were inadvertently introduced into the system are flushed into the spent dialysate. In the early years of the Y-set system, the tubing was rinsed with a hypochlorite disinfectant during bag exchange. Another advantage: patients do not have to carry a bag attached to their bodies.

The double (or twin)-bag system (Y-System with double bag) is similar to the Y-set system. Both bags in this system (the empty one and the one with the fresh solution) are connected to the tubing by the manufacturer and only one connection is required to be performed by the patient: that of the main limb with the catheter. The double-bag system is an improvement of the Y-system that eliminates a connection and further decreases the risk of infection [1-12].

In twelve randomized or quasi-randomized controlled trials with a total of 991 randomized patients comparing double-bag and/or Y-set CAPD exchange systems with standard systems, or comparing double-bag with Y-set systems, in patients with end-stage renal disease (ESRD) treated with CAPD; It was found that in trials comparing either the Y-set or double-bag systems with the standard systems, significantly fewer patients experienced peritonitis and the number of patient-months on CAPD per episode of peritonitis was consistently greater. When the double-bag systems were compared with the Y-set systems significantly fewer patients experienced peritonitis and the number of patient-months on CAPD per episode of peritonitis was also greater [1, 2].

In a multicenter, single-blinded, prospective randomized study on the use of a double-bag disconnect system (B) versus a Y-set disconnect system (Y). A total of 120 new end-stage renal failure patients were randomized: 60 each to the B and the Y systems. The patients were followed up for a median of 16 months. Peritonitis rates for the B and the Y systems were 33.5 and 29.4 patient-months per episode, respectively. Exit site infection rates for the B and Y systems were 17.4 and 16.0 patient-months per episode, respectively. Four catheters were removed in each group. Patients on the B system were hospitalized for 2.1 days per patient per year related to peritonitis and exit site infection, and those on the Y system were hospitalized for 1.2 days. There was no significant difference between the B and Y systems in the incidences of peritonitis (all causes and those due to coagulase-negative staphylococci), exit site infection, and in hospitalization days. However, there was a higher percentage of gram-positive infections in the Y system (52%) than in the B system (32%) and a lower percentage of gram-negative infections in the Y system (16%) than in the B system (32%). Patients on the B system had a better acceptance of the procedure than patients on the Y system, as assessed by a six-item, 10-point questionnaire. From this study, it is concluded that the B and Y systems are similar in the incidences of peritonitis and exit site infection, although the B system is better accepted by patients.

There is an accumulated experience evidence (level A) confirming that disconnecting (Y-set and double-bag) systems are superior to 'standard' systems regarding prevention of peritonitis. In particular, in eight randomized controlled trials (RCTs) or quasi-RCTs [4, 11], the Y-set delivery systems were compared with the 'standard' systems. In all but one [13] of the studies, the number of patients who experienced at least one episode of peritonitis was significantly less for patients using the Y-set compared with those on the 'standard' system. All the studies showed a significant increase in the number of months in between each episode of peritonitis. Also, in two controlled studies [11, 13] where the 'standard' system was compared with the double-bag systems, the results showed a significantly reduced incidence of peritonitis with the latter systems. Finally, in four controlled studies [2, 3, 8, 14], where the two newer methods, i.e. the Y-set and the double-bag systems, were compared, significantly fewer patients using the double-bag system experienced peritonitis.

In one prospective non-randomized study [15], patients were assigned to different CAPD disconnecting (Y-set, automated peritoneal dialysis) or non-disconnecting systems (spike, UV connection device) according to clinical and lifestyle criteria. Peritonitis rates were significantly less for disconnecting systems, but there was no difference in exit site infection rates. Two (evidence level B) studies showed no difference in peritonitis rates between UV-flash and disconnecting systems [16, 17]. One of them [16] additionally showed that the incidence of peritonitis of these two systems was significantly less than that of the 'standard' system. The length of the branches of the Y-set systems, in one study [18], was not related to the incidence of peritonitis.

Delivery systems and exit site infection. In seven RCTs, the incidence of exit site or tunnel infection is not significantly affected by the delivery system. In particular, four studies comparing the Y-set with the 'standard' system [7-10], two studies comparing the double-bag with the Y-set [3, 14] and one study comparing the double-bag with the 'standard' system [13] demonstrated no significant difference either in the number of patients who experienced exit site or tunnel infections, or in the number of patient-months on CAPD per episode of exit site infection. Guideline C. Disinfecting devices Disinfecting devices such as UV-flash [16,17], as well as microwave moist-heat [19] and xenon-based UV light, although effective in vitro [20], have not demonstrated improvement of peritonitis rates obtained by disconnecting systems. The results of the study by Kubey et al. [21], who quantified bacterial removal in Y-set and double-bag systems, emphasize the importance of the design of the fluid path flow (flush before fill) in the overall safe performance of these peritoneal dialysis systems.

A new, safe and convenient 5-L dual-chamber container for automated peritoneal dialysis

To further improve patient convenience and reduce the probability of infusing only the buffer contents from the outflow chamber, a new, safe and convenient 5-L dual-chamber container for automated peritoneal dialysis was designed. A 5-L dual-chamber container system with a dual-seal system consisting of a long seal between the dextrose chamber and buffer chambers and a short Safety Moon™ seal between the buffer chamber and container outflow connector. The safety and effectiveness of this new container system was assessed in a non-interventional, prospective, open-label, multi-centre, uncontrolled, Baxter-sponsored post-authorization safety study in 249 patients from 7 countries in Europe. No mis-infusion events were noted throughout the study where 68 519 Physioneal™ 5-L bags in Clear-Flex™ were used for an average (SD) of 4.3 (1.9) months per patient. Overall, the percentage of patients and/or care providers rating the 5-L bag preparation as very easy or easy at baseline (0-8 weeks), 9-16, 17-24 and 25-32 weeks ranged from 94 to 97%. Assuming a Poisson distribution for the bag count data, the estimated change in number of bicarbonate/lactate dialysis fluid bags (5 or 2.5 L) as a percent of prior bag use was -36%, while the estimated change in number of bags for ALL solutions as a percent of prior bag use was -31%. The predominant reasons given by the investigators for prescribing 5-L PD solutions at study onset were biocompatibility, easier and convenient for their patients to use, physiological pH and less bag connections. None of the 92 serious adverse events were suspected to be related to the Physioneal 5-L PD solution. The use of a larger, Physioneal 5-L bag mitigates the concern regarding the possibility of mis-infusing the buffer chamber solution, is convenient to use by the patient/health care provider and was associated with more than a 30% reduction in the weekly number of dialysis solution bags required per patient for their APD therapy[22].

A new twist lock connectology

The DextroLyte II (Dex II) Peritoneal Dialysis System was designed to improve safety and convenience in dialysis therapy. Connectors introduced with this system have a threaded recessed male connector with a corresponding female counterpart. Products are provided for CAPD, Single Use Y, Long Life Y and CCPD. Safety and convenience features intended to reduce peritonitis rates and improve patient acceptance include the following:

1. Connectors with threaded male and corresponding female counterparts which provide a dual seal
2. Easy-to-break frangible which seals the solution bag until ready for use
3. A flange on the connector ensures proper hand placement by providing a safety shield to prevent contamination during connection
4. A hinged shield containing an impregnated povidone-iodine sponge easily snaps around the bag connector
5. A Quick Disconnect Clamp (QDC) provides external occlusion permitting safe disconnection for bagless techniques without opening the system
6. A standard medication port provides easy access for administration of intraperitoneal medication.

A multicenter study performed in nine centers with total patient participants 121 and total patient months 1207. Overall peritonitis rate was 1 episode in 43 patient months The Dex II peritoneal dialysis systems was claimed to provide safe dialysis therapy as evidenced by the exceptional peritonitis rates. Patient acceptance has been excellent due to the inclusion of the safety and convenience features described [23].

REFERENCES

[1] Daly, CD; Campbell, MK; MacLeod, AM; et al. Do the T-set and double-bag systems reduce the incidence of CAPD peritonitis? *Nephrol Dial Transplant* 2001; 16: 341–347

[2] Kiernan, L; Kliger, A; Gorban-Brennan, N; et al. Comparison of continuous ambulatory peritoneal dialysis-related infections with different ''T-tubing'' exchange systems. *J Am Soc Nephrol* 1995; 5: 1835–1838.

[3] Li, PK; Szeto, CC, Law, MC; et al. Comparison of double-bag and Y-set disconnect systems in continuous ambulatory peritoneal dialysis: a randomized prospective multicenter study. *Am J Kidney Dis*. 1999; 33(3):535-40.

[4] Maiorca, R; Cantaluppi, A; Cancarini, GC; et al. Prospective controlled trial of a Y-connector and disinfectant to prevent peritonitis in continuous ambulatory peritoneal dialysis. *Lancet* 1983; 2: 642–644.

[5] Rottembourg, J; Brouard, R; Issad, I; et al. Pre´vention des peritonites au cours de la dialyse pe´ritone´ale c¸ontinue ambulatoire. Intere^ t des syste`mes deconnectables. *Presse Med* 1988; 17: 1349–1353.

[6] Lindholm, T; Simonsen, O; Krutzen, L; et al. Evaluation of a new take-off system: a prospective randomized multicenter study.*Adv Perit Dial* 1988; 4: 264–265.

[7] Churchill, DN; Taylor, DW; Vas, SI; et al. (for the Canadian CAPD Clinical Trials Group). Peritonitis in continuous ambulatory peritoneal dialysis (CAPD): a multi-center randomized clinical trial comparing the Y connector disinfectant system to standard systems. *Perit Dial Int* 1989; 9: 159–163.

[8] Owen, JE; Walker, RG; Lemon, J; et al. Randomized study of peritonitis with conventional versus O-set techniques in continuous ambulatory peritoneal dialysis. *Perit Dial Int* 1992; 12: 216–220.

[9] Cheng, IK; Chan, CY; Cheng, SW; et al. A randomized prospective study of the cost effectiveness of the conventional spike, O-set, and UVXD techniques in continuous ambulatory peritoneal dialysis. *Perit Dial Int* 1994; 14: 255–260.

[10] Li, PKT; Chan, TH; So WY; et al.Comparison of Y-set disconnect system (Ultraset) versus conventional spike system in uremic patients on CAPD: outcome and cost analysis. *Perit Dial Int* 1996; 16 [Suppl 1]:S368–S370.

[11] Monteon, F; Correa-Rotter, R; Paniagua, R; et al. Prevention of peritonitis with disconnect systems in CAPD: a randomized controlled trial. *Kidney Int* 1998; 54: 2123–2128.

[12] Buoncristiani U. Birth and evolution of the "Y" set. ASAIO J. 1996; 42(1):8-11.

[13] Dryden, MS; McCann, M; Wing, AJ; Phillips, I. Controlled trial of a Y-set dialysis delivery system to prevent peritonitis in patients receiving continuous ambulatory peritoneal dialysis. *J Hosp Infect* 1992; 20: 185–192.

[14] Harris, DCH; Yuill ,EJ; Byth ,K;Chapman, JR; Hunt, C. Twin versus single-bag disconnect systems: infection rates and cost of continuous ambulatory peritoneal dialysis. *J Am Soc Nephrol* 1996; 7: 2392–2398.

[15] Burkart ,JM; Jordan, JR; Durnell, TA; Case, LD. Comparison of exit-site infections in disconnect versus nondisconnect systems for peritoneal dialysis. *Perit Dial Int* 1992; 12: 317–320.

[16] Nakamura, Y; Hara, Y; Ishida, H; Morikawi, K; Shigemoto, K. A randomized multicenter trial to evaluate the effects of UV-flash system on peritonitis rates in CAPD. *Adv Perit Dial* 1992; 8: 313–315.

[17] Bailie, GR; Rasmussen, R; Hollister, A; Eisele, G. Incidence of CAPD peritonitis in patients using UVXD or O-set systems. *Clin Nephrol* 1990; 33: 252–254.

[18] Viglino, G; Colombo, A; Scalamogna, A et al. Prospected randomized study of two Y-devices in continuous ambulatory peritoneal dialysis. *Perit Dial Int* 1989; 9: 165–168.

[19] Fessia, SL; Grabowy, RS; Bousquet, GG. Effectiveness of microwave moist-heat intraluminal disinfection on CAPD connectology. *Adv Perit Dial* 1991; 7: 204–207.

[20] Kubey, W; Holmes, CJ. In vitro studies of the microbicidal effectiveness of a xenon-based ultraviolet light in continuous ambulatory peritoneal dialysis connections. *Blood Purif* 1991; 9: 102–108.

[21] Kubey W, Straka P, Holmes CJ. Importance of product design on effective bacterial removal by fluid convection in Y-set and twin-bag systems. Blood Purif 1998; 16: 154–161.

[22] Povlsen, JV; Koch, M; Eklund, B; et al. A new, safe and convenient 5-L dual-chamber container for automated peritoneal dialysis**.** Nephrol Dial Transplant. 2011; 26(1):299-303.

[23] Fox, K; Adcock, A; Raymon, K; Walker, P.Analysis of clinical experience with a new twist lock connectology. *Adv Perit Dial.* 1992; 8:291-3.

PHARMACOLOGIC ADVANCES

Peritoneal fibrosis and peritoneal sclerosis represent some of the most disastrous complications of PD. Favorable results have been obtained with tamoxifen for similar conditions such as retroperitoneal fibrosis. Therefore, the use of tamoxifen has been suggested in peritoneal fibrosis and peritoneal sclerosis associated with dialysis [1]. Tamoxifen inhibits protein kinas C, a mediator of cellular proliferation; it probably inhibits other growth factors (epidermal growth factor and calmodulin) as well.

Del Peso et al. recently reported their experience with 23 patients diagnosed with peritoneal sclerosis [2]. Nine of the patients were treated with tamoxifen for an average of 15 months; 14 were not treated. Four of the untreated patients developed encapsulating peritoneal sclerosis, but none of the treated patients did. The overall mortality for the untreated group was 71%; it was 22% for those who were treated ($p = 0.03$). These encouraging results and the poor prognosis associated with peritoneal sclerosis should stimulate further studies on the beneficial effects of tamoxifen in the prevention and resolution of peritoneal fibrosis.

Sodium sulfite has been shown to suppress methylglyoxal-induced hypervascularity, AGE formation, and other macroscopic alterations in the peritoneum. Pimagedine has also been shown to inhibit formation of AGEs and to slow the progression of nephropathy in animal models [3, 4]. The potential use of potent antioxidants, AGE inhibitors, and AGE breakers as salvage therapy for peritoneal membrane failure should be considered.

Many patients treated with continuous ambulatory peritoneal dialysis (CAPD) need antihypertensive agents such as calcium antagonists, which produce reflex tachycardia through activation of the sympathetic nervous system [5, 6.7]. In CAPD, blood pressure control depends on peritoneal ultrafiltration and a decline in fluid retention [8, 9]. Therapy with anti-hypertensive drugs is indicated primarily in the few patients in whom hypertension persists despite seemingly adequate volume control. Elevated blood pressure can usually be controlled by most classes of antihypertensive agents. Several large-scale clinical studies [10, 11], suggested that angiotensin converting enzyme (ACE) inhibitors and angiotensin type II receptor blockers (ARBs) can be used in patients with renal disease. However, these agents are more effective in reducing blood pressure when volume is depleted or salt is restricted [12, 13]. In CAPD patients, volume expansion plays an important role in both the development and maintenance of hypertension [7]. Thus ACE inhibitors and angiotensin type II receptor blockers (ARBs) are less effective than calcium antagonists, which are very effective and well tolerated in these patients [14].

Azelnidipine, a newly developed calcium antagonist, has unique characteristics in that it causes less reflex stimulation of the sympathetic nervous system [15]. A crossover method was used to compare the effects of amlodipine (5 – 10 mg daily) and azelnidipine (8 – 16 mg daily) on drain volume and weekly creatinine clearance in 9 CAPD patients. Each calcium antagonist was administered for 3 months and then switched for the other. As compared with amlodipine, azelnidipine increased drain volume by 13% ± 2% ($p < 0.05$) and weekly creatinine clearance by 12% ± 2% ($p < 0.05$). No significant differences in blood pressure and urine volume were observed. The increases in drain volume produced by azelnidipine resulted from less activation of the sympathetic nervous system. The activation of the sympathetic nervous system induced by calcium antagonists may be important in the regulation of drain volume in CAPD patients [16].

References

[1] Diaz-Buxo, JA. Peritoneal sclerosis in a woman on continuous cyclic peritoneal dialysis. *Semin Dial* 1992; 5:317–20.

[2] del Peso, G; Bajom, MA; Gil, F; *et al.* Clinical experience with tamoxifen in peritoneal fibrosing syndromes.*Adv Perit Dial* 2003; 19:32–5.

[3] Nakayama, M;Sakai, A; Numata, M; Hosoya, T. Hyper-vascular change and formation of advanced glycation end products in the peritoneum caused by methylglyoxal and the effect of an anti-oxidant, sodium sulfite. *Am J Nephrol* 2003; 23:390–4.

[4] Bolton, WK; Cattran, DC; Williams, ME; *et al.* Randomized trial of an inhibitor of formation of advanced glycation end products in diabetic nephropathy. *Am J Nephrol* 2004; 24:32–40.

[5] Collins, AJ; Kasiske, B; Herzog, C; *et al.*, for the United States Renal Data System. Excerpts from the United States Renal Data System 2004 annual data report: atlas of end-stage renal disease in the United States. *Am J Kidney Dis* 2005; 45(Suppl 1):A5–7.

[6] Patient Registration Committee, Japanese Society for Dialysis Therapy. The current state of chronic dialysis treatment in Japan. *J Jpn Soc Dial Ther* 2002; 35:1155–84.

[7] Mailloux, LU; Haley, WE. Hypertension in the ESRD patient: pathophysiology, therapy, outcomes, and future directions. *Am J Kidney Dis* 1998; 32:705–19.

[8] Wang, X; Axelsson, J; Lindholm, B; Wang, T. Volume status and blood pressure in continuous ambulatory peritoneal dialysis patients. *Blood Purif* 2005; 23:373–8.

[9] Menon, MK; Naimark, DM; Bargman, JM; Vas, SI; Oreopoulos, DG. Long-term blood pressure control in a cohort of peritoneal dialysis patients and its association with residual renal function. Nephrol Dial Transplant 2001; 16:2207–13.
[10] The GISEN (Gruppo Italiano di Studi Epidemiologici in Nefrologia) group. Randomised placebo-controlled trial of effect of ramipril on decline in glomerular filtration rate and risk of terminal renal failure in proteinuric, non-diabetic nephropathy. Lancet 1997; 349:1857–67.
[11] Brenner, B; Cooper, ME; de Zeeuw; D; et al, for the RENAAL Study investigators. Effects of losartan on renal and cardiovascular outcomes in patients with type 2 diabetes and nephropathy. N Engl J Med 2001; 345:861–9.
[12] Griffiths, CD; Morgan, TO; Delbridge, LM. Effects of combined administration of ACE inhibitor and angiotensin II receptor antagonist are prevented by a high NaCl intake. J Hypertens 2001; 19:2087–95.
[13] Wing, LM; Arnolda, LF; Harvey, PJ; et al. Low-dose diuretic and/or dietary sodium restriction when blood pressure is resistant to ACE inhibitor. *Blood Press* 1998; 7:299–307.
[14] London, GM; Marchais, SJ; Guerin, AP; et al. Salt and water retention and calcium blockade in uremia. Circulation1990; 82:105–13.
[15] Wellington K, Scott LJ. Azelnidipine. Drugs 2003; 63:2613–21, 2623–4.
[16] Suzuki; Inoue, T; Kobayashi, K; Shoda, J; Nakamoto, H. The Newly Developed Calcium Antagonist, Azelnidipine, Increases Drain Volume in Continuous Ambulatory Peritoneal Dialysis Patients. *Adv Perit Dial* 2006; 22:18-23.

PERITONEAL DIALYSIS: ADVANCES IN THE DEVELOPING WORLD

Chronic peritoneal dialysis is widely available in industrialized countries. In developing countries it is not uniformly available, so patient management often relies on conservative measures and intermittent peritoneal dialysis (IPD) [1, 2, 3, 4]. However, ESRD patients treated in such a way may die from uremia and complications of IPD [3, 4, 5, 6, 7].Probably the most important breakthrough in peritoneal dialysis in the developing world was the reduction in the need of frequent IPD with use of a new approach combining conservative measures and the urea lowering effect of acacia gum (AG) supplementation [7-15].

In one study, six patients with ESRD and significant uremia that required at least one IPD session to maintain life were enrolled in a clinical trial investigating the use of acacia gum supplementation to improve wellbeing and providing patients with ESRD significant reduction in the frequency of IPD sessions [7]**:** Three patients aged between 11-13 years (each with, oxalosis, cystinosis, and ESRD of undetermined etiology) and have symptomatic uremia required at least one peritoneal dialysis despite low-protein diet and other conservative measures of ESRD, they had no reductions in urine output nor edema and were normotensive, their pre -dialysis creatinine clearance was less than 5 ml/min by a formula developed by Cock and Gault [16] were treated with this new approach. One patient complied with the protocol for only 10 days and died after 6 months despite intermittent peritoneal dialysis. Two patients completed one year on this therapeutic regimen. Both patients reported improved wellbeing. Neither became acidotic or uremic, and neither required dialysis during the one year of the study period. Both patients maintained serum creatinine and urea levels not previously achieved without dialysis. The other three patients were managed with IPD; all died with in less than 6 months [7].Of the 2 surviving patients on AG supplementation, one patient stopped AG supplementation after one year and died within one month despite IPD. The other patient continued to be treated with this novel therapy and continued to experience improved wellbeing and dialysis freedom during 6 completed years [6, 15].The other three patients observed all died while they were managed with IPD.Figure-1 shows the survival of the patients treated with AG supplementation compared to patients treated with IPD alone. Dietary proteins in the enrolled patients were restricted to 1 g/kg/day with at least 50% of the total intake given as egg albumin. Protein and phosphorus restriction was primarily achieved by restricting meat, poultry, fish, milk, cheese, and yogurt. Powder AG (1g/kg/day in 2-3 divided doses diluted with desired amounts of water with or without the addition of sugar and juices).Many of the conservative measures used with acacia gum such as high calorie diet, water soluble vitamins, calcium carbonate supplements, and erythropoietin are also necessary in patients treated by dialysis [17-24].

In a series of 80 patients with CRF, 14 (16.5%) patients were treated with the new approach using the urea lowering effect of acacia gum supplementation plus the traditional conservative measures .Treatment resulted in amelioration of the uremic symptoms and lowering of blood urea levels and delaying the need for dialysis. In this sample of 80 patients the longest survival of 5 years was achieved in 2 patients, both treated initially with IPD

One of them was transplanted and the other was treated with combination of the traditional conservative measures and acacia gum supplementation[14,25].

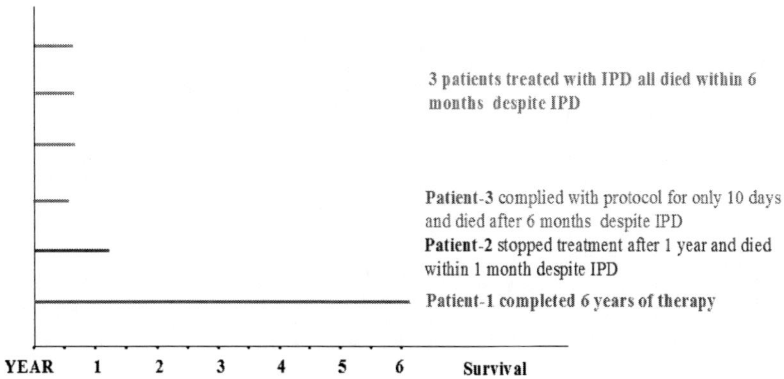

Figure 1. shows the survival of the patients treated with AG supplementation compared to patients treated with IPD alone. (Please provide a name for Y-axis).

The main principles and concepts supporting this important breakthrough are:

1. The fact that a patient with CRF may remain asymptomatic and to a large extent successful in maintaining normal body composition despite a reduction in the GFR over 80 % ,suggests that there could be a possible intervention to bring back the patient to the asymptomatic state and reducing the frequency of IPD[26].
2. With appropriate dietary and pharmacologic management, patients with non-terminal CRF can be maintained surprisingly well [8,27] and the transition from non-terminal CRF to ESRF represents a small decrement of renal function resulting in a large physiologic hurdle for the patient[28].The addition to these effective traditional measures, an agent enhance fecal nitrogen excretion can possibly bridge this gap resulting from this small decrement of renal function and markedly reducing the need for IPD.

REFERENCES

[1] Ehlayelm, MS; Akl, KF. Childhood chronic renal failure in Qatar. Br. J. Clin. Pract 1992; 46, 19–20.

[2] El-Reshaid, K; Madan, MK; Naryanan Nampoory, MR; EL-Reshaid, W; Johny, KV. Pediatric dialysis and transplantation in Kuwait over the past 11 years. Pediatr. Nephrol. 1999; 13, 259–264.

[3] Madani, K; Outkesh, H; Rastegar A, Van Why, S. Chronic renal failure in Iranian children. Pediatr. Nephrol.2001; 16, 140–144.

[4] Barrat, TM; Griefer, I. Pediatric nephrology around the world, Overview. In: Pediatric Nephrology. 4th ed. Barrat TM, Avner ED, Harmon WE. Lippincott Williams and Wilkins, Baltimore, MD, USA, 1349–1372; 1999.

[5] Al Mosawi, AJ. The etiology of chronic renal failure in 54 Iraqi children. Pediatr. Nephrol.2002; 463–464 .9. Al-Mosawi AJ. The challenge of chronic renal failure in the developing world. Possible use of acacia gum. Pediatr. Nephrol.2002; 63–464.

[6] Al Mosawi, AJ. 'The use of acacia gum in end stage renal failure.J Trop Pediatr. 2007; 53(5):362-5.

[7] Al-Mosawi, AJ. Acacia gum supplementation of a low-protein diet in children with end-stage renal disease.Pediatr Nephrol. 2004; 19(10):1156-9.

[8] Al Mosawi, AJ. Acacia gum therapeutic potential: possible role in the management of uremia – a new potential medicine. Therapy 2006; 3(2) 301-321.

[9] Al Mosawi, AJ. Comprehensive conservative management of ESRF: three –year dialysis freedom. Pediatr Nephrol 2006; 21(10): 1600.1601. (Abstracts: The 40th annual meeting of the ESPN October 7-10 Palermo Italy www.espn2006.org).

[10] Al Mosawi, AJ. A comprehensive conservative management for end-stage renal failure European Journal of Pediatrics. Volume 165, Supplement 1 / November, 2006 : 1-389 (Abstracts: European Academy of Pediatrics 2006-10-07 - 2006-10-10 Barcelona, Spain

[11] www.kenes.com/europaediatrics/).

[12] Mosawi, AJ. Continuous renal replacement in the developing world: Is there any alternative. Therapy (London) 2006:3(2): 265-272.

[13] Al Mosawi, AJ. Continuous renal replacement (CRRT) in the developing world: Is there any alternative? Pediatr Nephrol 2006; 21(3): 452. (Abstracts: Fourth International Conference on Pediatric Continuous Renal Replacement Therapy 24-25 February 2006 Zurich Switzerland.

[14] Al Mosawi, AJ. A Beneficial Effect of Acacia Gum in a Patient with Nephropathic Cystinosis and Chronic Renal Failure Pediatr Nephrol 2007; 22 (9):1401-1650. (Abstracts: 14 th Congress of the International Pediatric Nephrology Association 2006-08-31 - 2007-09-04 Budapest, Hungary

[15] www.ipna2007.com/final_programme/index.html).

[16] Al Mosawi, AJ. Renal Failure (CRF): An extra-ordinary experience. Pediatr Nephrol 2007; 22 (12):2151-2175 (Abstracts: Neprokids-WCN 07 Satellite symposium on Pediatric nephro-urological diseases April 27-April 29 Brazil).

[17] Al Mosawi, AJ. Six-year dialysis freedom in end-stage renal disease. Clin Exp Nephrol. 2009; 13 (5): 446-500.

[18] Zawad ET Jr.In Indications for dialysis. I: DaugirdasJt, Ing TS (Eds) Handbook of dialysis. Little Brown, Boston 3-7; 1988.

[19] Gruppe, WE; Harmon, WE; Spinozzi, NS.Protein and energy requirements in children receiving chronic hemodialysis. Kidney Int 1983; 24: S6-S10.

[20] Slatopolsky, E; Weerts, C; Lopez Hilkers; etal .Calcium carbonate as a phosphate binder in patients with chronic renal failure undergoing dialysis. N Engl J Med 1986); 315: 157-161.

[21] Anderoil, SP; Dunson, JW; Bergstein, JM .Calcium carbonate is an effective phosphorus binder in children with chronic renal failure Am J Kidney Dis 1987; 9: 206-210.

[22] Kriley, M; Warady, BA .Vitamins status of pediatric patients receiving long term peritoneal dialysis Am J clin Nutr 1991; 531: 1476-1479.

[23] Salusky, IB.Nutritional management of pediatric patients on chronic dialysis. In: Clinical Dialysis. Nissenson AR, Fine RN Gentile DE eds. Norwalk CT, Appleton & Lange, 535-548(1995).

[24] Warady, BA; Jabs, K. New hormones in the therapeutic arsenal of chronic renal failure: growth hormone and erythropoietin. Pediatr Clin N Am 1995; 42: 1551-1577.

[25] Jabs, K; Harmon, WE. Recombinant human erythropoietin therapy in children on dialysis. Adv Ren Replace Ther1996; 3: 24-36.

[26] Rigden, SP; Montini, G; Morris M; etal. Recombinant human erythropoietin therapy in children maintained by hemodialysis Pediatr Nephrol 1990; 4: 618-622.

[27] Al Mosawi, AJ .Chronic renal failure in Iraqi children: 14 year experience of a single center Journal of Nephrology and Renal Transplantation (JNRT). JNRT 1(1) 2008: 32 – 40.

[28] Briker, NS. The pathogenesis of the uremic state: "The trade –off hypothesis" N Engl J Med 1972; 286 1093-1099.

[29] Shoeneman, M. Dietary and pharmacologic treatment of chronic renal failure. In: Pediatric Kidney Disease. Edelmann CM ed., Little, Brown and Co. Boston, 475-487(1978).

[30] Harmon, WE. Chronic renal failure, Overview of chronic renal failure. In: Pediatric Nephrology. 4 th ed., Barrat TM, Avner ED, Harmon WE. Lippincott Williams and Wilkins, Baltimore, 1151-1154; 1999.

CONCLUSION

The objective of modern PD is to extent its initial survival advantage to long-term treatment. Recent advances in knowledge of mechanisms and new dialysis solutions are likely to make this possible. Technologic advances in PD could have an important impact on patient care. Recent advances in knowledge of mechanisms and new dialysis solutions are likely to make this possible. Advances on the modality including the use of icodextrine, automated PD, low-glucose degradation products, new solutions and individualized schedules promise to improve the prognosis of risk patients under dialysis such as diabetics and patients with congestive heart failure, the elderly, the fast transporters or the anuric.The success of peritoneal dialysis on the short-term is mainly dependent on the prevention of infectious and technical complications. The mid-term results will to a large extent be determined by the ability to remove enough uremic toxins to prevent uremic complications and malnutrition. The long-term challenge is the prevention of the development of structural abnormalities of the peritoneum leading to ultrafiltration failure and sometimes peritoneal sclerosis.

Improved efficacy and safety of peritoneal dialysis on the midterm can be achieved by individualization of the dialysis prescription taking residual renal function especially into account. Early start of dialysis might reduce the progression rate of renal function deterioration, but exposes the peritoneum to bio-incompatible dialysis solutions for a longer time. The long-term alterations in the peritoneal membrane are probably mainly caused by the continuous exposure to dialysis fluids, especially glucose, and perhaps the combination of low pH with lactate. The implications of long-term continuous ambulatory peritoneal dialysis using only more biocompatible dialysis fluids are not clear. To improve the efficacy and safety of peritoneal dialysis, careful monitoring of patients and dialysis is mandatory. This should include 24-hour urine collections and 24-hour dialysate collections to calculate the residual glomerular filtration rate and adequacy parameters. A peritoneal membrane function test should be done regularly with 3.86% glucose dialysate, including determinations of dialysate Na^+ and cancer antigen 125 to detect patients who are at risk for the development of structural abnormalities of the peritoneum.

In: Peritoneal Dialysis
Editors: A. Agarwal, L. Salman et al.
ISBN: 978-1-62257-896-2

Chapter 3

PERITONEAL TRANSPORT STATUS: A RISK FACTOR FOR PERITONEAL DIALYSIS

Bhadran Bose, Sunil V. Badve and David W. Johnson
Princess Alexandra Hospital,
Brisbane, Australia

ABSTRACT

The peritoneal membrane is the lifeline for peritoneal dialysis (PD) patients. Our understanding of mechanisms of injury and functional responses continues to expand and will hopefully lead to therapies that improve clinical outcomes. A key characteristic of the peritoneal membrane is its permeability or transport status. This can be measured by a variety of methods, but most commonly involves measurement of the ratio of dialysate to plasma concentration of creatinine following a 4 hour dwell of 2 L of 2.5% glucose dialysate (D:P Cr) using a Peritoneal Equilibration Test. Standardisation of the PET is critically important as the D:P Cr result can be appreciably influenced by a number of variables, including dialysate composition and volume, the presence or absence of a dialysate exchange preceding the PET and the proximity of the PET to dialysis commencement. Transport status is typically categorised into 4 groups according to the mean ± 1 standard deviation of D:P Cr: High (D:P Cr ≥0.81, 16%), High-average (D:P Cr 0.65-0.80, 51%), Low-average (D:P Cr 0.50-0.64, 28%), and Low (D:P Cr <0.50, 5%). Higher peritoneal transport status at the commencement of PD is independently associated with racial origin, older age and lower body mass index and predicts higher risks of both technique failure and death. We have also demonstrated that transport status can change significantly over time in an appreciable minority of patients and is associated with increased risks of encapsulating peritoneal sclerosis, membrane failure and death. High transporters on chronic PD are challenged by increased protein losses, high glucose absorption, and poor ultrafiltration. Treatment with automated PD has been associated with improved survival in high transporters and reduced survival in low transporters. Icodextrin may also provide ultrafiltration benefits in high transporters.

This chapter reviews in detail the assessment, diagnosis, predictors, prognostic implications and therapeutic management of peritoneal transport status in PD patients. Suggestions for future research directions are also discussed.

1. INTRODUCTION

Peritoneal dialysis (PD) is a well-established treatment of end stage kidney disease, which requires solute and fluid exchange across the peritoneal membrane between peritoneal capillary blood and a dialysis solution in the peritoneal cavity. The peritoneal membrane, consisting of the vascular wall, interstitium, mesothelium and adjacent fluid films, is a lifeline for PD patients. Our understanding of mechanisms of injury and functional responses of the peritoneal membrane continues to expand and will hopefully lead to therapies that improve clinical outcomes [1]. A key characteristic of the peritoneal membrane is its permeability or transport status. Several studies have examined the relationship between peritoneal membrane transport status and PD patient morbidity and mortality [2-6]. In this chapter, we have discussed the assessment, the diagnosis, the predictors, prognostic implication and therapeutic management of peritoneal membrane transport status in PD patients.

2. Assessment of Peritoneal Membrane Transport Status

The transport properties of the peritoneal membrane can be measured to characterise its functional status. A patient's membrane transport status can be evaluated by different methods, such as the peritoneal equilibration test (PET), the personal dialysis capacity test (PDC) and the mini-PET test (Table 1).

2.1. Peritoneal Equilibration Test

The PET was introduced by Twardowski in 1987 [7] and is the standard method for evaluating peritoneal transport characteristics in PD patients. It is a semiquantitative assessment of peritoneal membrane transport function. The standardized test for clinical utility measures dialysate creatinine and glucose levels at 0, 2 and 4 hours of dwell and serum levels of creatinine and glucose at any time during the test. The most common parameters examined are the dialysate:plasma creatinine ratio at 4 hours (D:P Cr 4h) and the ratio of 4 hour dialysate glucose to initial dialysate glucose concentration ($D:D_0$).

The standard four-hour PET consists of the following steps:

1. The exchange preceding the equilibration test must dwell for 8-12 hours.
2. The pretest exchange is completely drained over 20 minutes in the sitting position (drain not to exceed 25 minutes).
3. A blood sample is collected at the end of drainage.
4. A sample of dialysis solution is obtained from the test bag to be infused and a 2 L of 2.5% dialysis solution is infused in portions of 400 ml per 2 min over a total of 10 min. The patient is in the supine position during the infusion and rolls from side to side after each 400 ml is infused for better mixing of residual volume and infused solution.
5. Exactly 10 min after the start of infusion, at the completion infusion (0 dwell time), 200 ml of solution is drained into the bag, mix well, a 10 ml sample of dialysate is taken and the remaining 190 ml reinfused. The patient is ambulatory during the dwell period.
6. Samples of dialysate are taken with the same technique after 30 min, 60 min, 120 min, and 180 min of dwell time.

7. After a 4-hour dwell time, the dialysate is drained over 20 min with the patient in the sitting position, total volume is measured and a sample is taken.
8. The total time of the equilibration exchange is 270 min.
9. A blood sample is obtained at the end of drainage.
10. All the samples are sent for solute measurement (creatinine, urea and glucose).
11. The D/D_0 glucose and the D:P ratios for creatinine, urea, electrolytes, phosphates and proteins are measured.

After commencing PD, the initial PET is best performed after the first 4 weeks, since peritoneal permeability appears to increase during the first 2-4 weeks. PETs performed within first month of initiating PD may be relatively inaccurate [8].

Table 1. Different peritoneal function tests Advantages and Disadvantages

Tests	Advantages	Disadvantages
Original PET	Categories high/average/low transporter and guides prescription Widely Used Defines UF failure	No information on sodium sieving, FWT or OC
PDC	More reliable data because of measuring points Estimates net peritoneal fluid loss (peritoneal reabsorption) Computer-aided prescription	Multiple laboratory tests needed. Software support for calculation needed.
Mini-PET	Measures FWT Lasts only 1 hour	Small solute transport difficult to interpret No information on OC or peritoneal reabsorption
Double mini PET	Measures FWT and OC Lasts only 2 hours	Small solute transport difficult to interpret No information on OC or peritoneal reabsorption

FWT – Free Water Transport; OC – osmotic conductance

The advantages and disadvantages of the PET are listed in Table 1. The PET is the most commonly performed evaluation of peritoneal transport status because it is easy to perform, the standard values are well established and it does not require any complicated calculations. It also helps to define ultrafiltration (UF) failure and categorises the membrane as high/high-average/low-average/low, which guides prescription. The downside is that the D:P and D/D_0 results are rather sensitive to laboratory errors and there is no information provided by the PET on sodium sieving, free water transport and osmotic conductance.

2.2. Personal Dialysis Capacity

The PDC is another approach to assess peritoneal membrane status [9]. The test uses a computerized mathematical model based on the three-pore model to describe peritoneal transport characteristics. It uses data collected over five exchanges with different glucose strengths and dwell times. It describes the peritoneal membrane characteristics by means of three parameters.

The parameters are:

1. The surface area over diffusion distance (A0/dX), which represents the effective surface area available for diffusion and is roughly comparable with the mass transfer coefficient and the dialysate over plasma concentration ratio (D/P) value of the PET test.
2. The reabsorption parameter (JvR), which measures the reabsorption of fluid from the peritoneal cavity after the osmotic (glucose) gradient has dissipiated.
3. The large pore fluid flux (JvL), which determines the loss of protein to the PD fluid.

The PDC test is a robust and accurate method to describe the peritoneal membrane transport characteristics [12] and can estimate peritoneal reabsoprtion. However, its main drawbacks are that it requires multiple laboratory tests and software support for calculations. There are very few tests comparing the clinical uitility of the PET vs PDC. Van Biesen and colleagues compared the abilities of the PET versus PDC to discriminate inflammation as the cause of fast transport status in 135 incident PD patients [12]. They observed that only large pore flux (J(v)L), but not surface area over diffusion distance (A0/dX) or dialysate over plasma concentration (D:P Cr 4h), was related to C-reactive protein. Using multivariable Cox proportional hazards model analysis with adjustment for age, only higher PDC-determined was associated with mortality. They concluded that the combination of JvL and A0/dX allows much better discrimination of inflammation from anatomic constitution as a cause of an fast transport status than the PET-determined D:P Cr 4h. However, given the small sample size and single centre design, additional studies are required to confirm this finding.

2.3. Mini-PET

The Mini-PET is a simpler and less time consuming version of the PET, but is less popular due to flaws [9]. It is performed over 1 hour using hypertonic 3.86% glucose solution and represents a simple and fast method of assessing free water transport and ultrafiltration [10]. There is also a double mini-PET, which involves a combination of two consecutive 1-hour PETs with 1.36 and 3.86% glucose solutions, respectively. These tests provide calculation of free water transport, osmotic conductance for glucose as well as ultrafiltration through small pores. The double mini-PET is a simple and rapid test that is particularly useful; for evaluating patients with reduced ultrafiltration (UF) capacity [11].

3. Categorisation of Peritoneal Membrane Transport Status

Based on the results of the PET, PD patients are classified as low, low-average, high-average or high transporters, according to the results of an individual's measured D:P Cr 4h and/or D/D_0 glucose in relation to the population mean ± 1 standard deviation.

- **High transporter** - These patients, accounting for approximately 15% of PD patients, have the most rapid and complete equilibration of creatinine and urea. They rapidly lose their osmotic gradient for ultrafiltration because of dialysate glucose diffusion into the blood via the highly permeable membrane. They are defined by a D:P Cr greater than 1 SD above the mean, or a D/D_0 glucose of more than 1 SD below the mean.

- **High-average transporter** - These patients, accounting for approximately 50% of PD patients, are defined by a D:P Cr 4h between the mean and +1 SD or a D/Do glucose between the mean and -1 SD.
- **Average transporter** - These patients, accounting for approximately 30% of PD patients, are defined by a D:P Cr 4h between the mean and -1 SD or a D/D_0 glucose between the mean and +1 SD.
- **Low transporter** - These patients, accounting for approximately 5% of PD patients, have slower and less complete equilibration of urea and creatinine, reflecting low membrane permeability or small effective peritoneal surface area. They are defined by a D:P Cr less than 1 SD below the mean, or a D/D_0 glucose of more than 1 SD above the mean.

Table 2. Categorisation of peritoneal transport status

Transport Category	D:P Cr 4h	D/D_0 glucose
High	> 0.80	<0.26
High-average	0.65-0.80	0.26-0.38
Low-average	0.50-0.64	0.39-0.49
Low	<0.50	>0.49

Almost 90 percent of properly conducted PETs show consistency in both D:P Creatinine and D/D_0 glucose [13].

4. Predictors of Baseline Peritoneal Transport Status

Peritoneal permeability, as assessed by PET, varies widely between patients and has been shown to differ significantly between distinct populations [14]. The factors that predict peritoneal transport status in PD patients remain poorly understood [15]. Studies, which have attempted to address this question to date, have been conflicting and often limited by small numbers, highly selected patient populations and the inclusion of prevalent patients (thereby potentially introducing informative censoring bias).

The largest study in this area was published by Rumpsfeld and colleagues [16]. Their study characterized peritoneal transport in a large incident PD population in Australia and New Zealand using PET data obtained from the Australian and New Zealand Dialysis and Transplant Association (ANZDATA) Registry. They demonstrated that older age and Maori/Pacific Islander racial origin were significant independent predictors of high peritoneal transport status. Moreover, patients with a BMI exceeding 25 kg/m^2 were significantly less likely to be high transporters. These same relationships were observed when peritoneal transport was modeled as a continuous variable (D:P Cr 4h), except that higher D:P Cr 4h was also significantly associated with the presence of cerebrovascular disease. However, gender, hypertension, lung disease, coronary artery disease, peripheral vascular disease, prior renal transplantation, residual renal function, diabetes mellitus, smoking status and prior haemodialysis were not predictive of either increased peritoneal transport category or D:P Cr 4h.

One of the key new findings of this study was the observation of significant ethnic variation in peritoneal permeability characteristics. In Australian and New Zealand PD patients, the mean D:P Cr 4h (0.69±0.13) was approximately 0.04 higher than that found by Twardowski in a North American population [7] and was higher again in indigenous Australians and New Zealanders (0.70±0.14 and 0.71±0.13, respectively). On the other hand, the mean values for D:P Cr 4h were significantly lower in Asians (0.68±0.11) and Asian Indians (0.67±0.13) than in Caucasians (0.69±0.12). In keeping with this observation, Raj and colleagues who examined ethnic variability in PET measurements, observed that Oriental (Chinese and Polynesian) PD patients were less likely to be high transporters (16.7%) than either Caucasian (24.6%) or African-American patients (22%) [17]. Other studies in different PD patient populations have reported the proportion of high transporters to range from 15% in North and Latin Americans [3, 18] to 22% in African-Americans [17] to approximately 50% in Greeks [19] and Asian Indians [20].

These results differ from a sub-study of the CANUSA trial [3], in which baseline high peritoneal transport was not associated with racial origin, but was predicted by increasing age, male gender and diabetes mellitus in 606 North American PD patients. The disparity in results may be explained by the highly selected nature of the predominantly Caucasian subjects participating in the CANUSA trial compared with the unselected Registry population studied in the ANZDATA Registry Study. Alternatively, it is conceivable that the relationship between peritoneal transport and patient factors is population-specific.

Population differences may also at least partly explain the apparently conflicting observations regarding the influence of diabetes mellitus on peritoneal permeability, in which some studies have found a significant association between the two conditions [3, 15, 18, 21], whilst others have not [20, 22, 23]. Apart from diabetes mellitus, other comorbidities may contribute to high peritoneal small solute clearance at the commencement of PD. The ANZDATA Registry Study demonstrated that the presence of cerebrovascular disease was predictive of increased D:P Cr 4h on multiple linear regression, but just failed to reach statistical significance ($p=0.077$) in the multivariate ordinal logistic regression analysis. In a prospective, single centre cohort study of 303 patients commencing PD, Davies and colleagues observed that grade of comorbidity, (which included diabetes, vascular disease and malignancy), was significantly associated with increased solute transport [4]. The effect was not entirely explained by diabetes alone, as the total comorbidity load had an additional impact.

Since the effective peritoneal vascular surface area principally determines peritoneal permeability, it is possible that the associations identified between high transporter status and both older age and cerebrovascular disease may reflect underlying damage to the peritoneal vasculature. For example, Park and colleagues [24] observed that advanced glycosylation end products (AGE), which have been implicated in the atherosclerotic complications of uraemia [25] and ageing [26], were deposited to a greater extent in high transporters.

The observed relationship between solute transport and comorbidity at the start of treatment may also be due to associated inflammation and malnutrition, as part of the malnutrition, inflammation, atherosclerosis (MIA) syndrome [27]. The frequent occurrence of hypoalbuminaemia in high transporters has fuelled speculation that malnutrition may explain the apparent link between peritoneal transport, comorbidity and poorer clinical outcomes [1]. Although peritoneal protein losses are increased in high transporters [28], the association between D:P Cr 4h and lower serum albumin is present prior to the initiation of dialysis [1]. A study by Nolph and colleagues suggested a correlation between high peritoneal solute flux and impairment of nutritional parameters other than serum albumin [29], but this has not been shown in subsequent, larger studies [3, 30, 31]. Other investigators have suggested that the hypoalbuminaemia and adverse clinical outcomes frequently observed in high transporters may reflect a greater incidence of underlying chronic inflammation [32, 33]. However, some studies have failed to identify any significant relationship between inflammatory markers and D:P Cr 4h [34, 35].

It has also been suggested that uraemia per se and the duration of end-stage renal failure may affect peritoneal membrane structure and function, as well as the likelihood of comorbid disease burden [36]. Williams and coworkers observed that peritoneal vasculopathy and submesothelial fibrosis, which correlate with increased membrane solute transport, were already significantly increased in pre-dialysis and haemodialysis patients [37]. Moreover, Wilmer and associates noted that the risk of high transporter status was increased more than 2-fold on univariate analysis in 19 patients treated with PD after a failed renal transplant compared with PD patients without a history of prior renal transplantation (who presumably had a shorter cumulative duration of end-stage renal failure) [38].

Patients undergoing long-term treatment with CAPD develop permanent loss of UF. Heimburger and colleagues reported the risk of UF loss increased with time on CAPD 2.6% after one year and 30.9% after six years) and did not correlate with the incidence of peritonitis. Increased peritoneal transport of small solutes was observed in most patients with loss of UF, whereas the rate of protein transport was not increased. Loss of UF was in most cases associated with rapid glucose absorption and loss of the osmotic driving force, resulting in a low and short-lived net ultrafiltration [39].

5. Prognostic Implications

5.1. Peritoneal Transport Status

Although there are some conflicting studies, the bulk of evidence to date indicates that high peritoneal transport status is a risk factor for mortality, whilst low peritoneal transport status connotes a favourable prognosis. In an analysis of the CANUSA data, Churchill et al [40] demonstrated that the relative risk of either technique failure or death was increased by 19% (95% confidence limits 5% to 34%) for each 0.1 increase in D:P Cr 4h. Two-year survival probabilities of high, high-average, low-average and low transporters were 70.5%, 72.4%, 80.4% and 90.9%, respectively ($p=0.11$). The 2-year probabilities of both patient and technique survival were 48%, 52%, 61% and 86%, respectively ($p=0.006$). These results were observed despite the fact that small solute clearances were greater (although not significantly) with higher transport status. Fried et al similarly demonstrated in a prospective study of 123 PD patients that the respective 3-year survival probabilities of high, high-average, low-average and low transporters were 70.5%, 90.9%, 88.9% and

100% ($p<0.05$), despite no significant differences observed in small solute clearance between the groups [5]. Davies and associates prospectively analysed survival in 210 and subsequently 303 consecutive PD patients using Cox proportional hazards models and identified that a high D:P Cr 4h was an independent predictor of death [41]. Similar results were reported by Wu et al [22], Wang et al [6], Hung et al [23] and Cueto-Manzano et al [21] in population sizes ranging between 46 and 171.

However, more recent studies have failed to observe an independent relationship between peritoneal permeability and PD outcomes [42-45]. One of the well-known of these investigations was the ADEMEX trial, which observed no significant effect of baseline peritoneal transport characteristics (as determined by the dialysis adequacy and transport test) on the survival of 965 PD patients [43]. The apparent disparity in findings may be explained by the fact that the ADEMEX trial predominantly included prevalent patients, thereby potentially introducing informative censoring bias.

Similarly, the prospective, multicentre European Automated PD Outcome Study (EAPOS) found that baseline D:P Cr 4h had no effect on overall or technique survival in 177 patients [42]. However, the results may have been adversely affected by the preferential selection of anuric, prevalent automated PD patients and by the relatively low number (n=31) of deaths (thereby making a possible type 2 statistical error likely). Other negative studies [33, 44, 45] have likewise been limited by small sample sizes ($\leq$213 patients), short follow-up times, low event rates and restriction to single centre observations. There is also a possibility that racial differences influenced the relationship between peritoneal transport and outcomes. For example, a study by Chung and associates observed that D:P Cr 4h was an independent predictor of mortality in 136 Korean PD patients, but not in 106 Swedish PD patients [2]. These differences however may also have been attributable to centre effects (since they involved only 1 centre in Korea and another in Sweden), differences in PET protocols (4.25% versus 2.5% glucose monohydrate solutions), informative censoring bias due to a much higher transplantation rate in the Swedish centre, and inadequate statistical power.

The exact mechanisms for the poorer survival of high and high-average transporters remain uncertain, but may relate at least partially to impaired ultrafiltration and fluid overload [6, 33, 45-47]. High peritoneal transport is associated with a more rapid absorption of glucose and hence dissipation of the osmotic gradient required for sustained ultrafiltration. There is evidence that patients with symptomatic fluid retention are 3.7 times more likely to be high than low transporters [48]. It has also been argued that the increased mortality among high transporters is primarily due to an association between D:P Cr 4h and comorbid illness burden [4]. Chung and colleagues reported that high transport status was an independent risk factor for mortality in patients with comorbid disease, but not in those without comorbidity [49].

Malnutrition may also have contributed to the excess mortality in high transporters, since such patients have a higher prevalence of hypoalbuminaemia [1, 6, 18, 40]. A low serum albumin correlates with other markers of malnutrition, such as normalised protein catabolic rate and subjective global assessment [50], and is strongly predictive of PD patient death [51, 52].

A study performed by our group examined a large cohort of Australian and New Zealand PD patients using PET data obtained from the Australian and New Zealand Dialysis and Transplant Association (ANZDATA) Registry [16]. It demonstrated that peritoneal transport status is a highly significant risk factor for both mortality and death-censored technique failure in the Australian and New Zealand incident PD patient populations. This risk was independent of demographic characteristics, BMI, comorbid clinical illnesses, peritoneal small solute clearances and residual renal function. Moreover, peritoneal permeability remained a risk factor for adverse PD outcomes regardless of whether it is analysed as a continuous or categorical variable. The study looked at 5170 individuals who began PD treatment between 1999 and 2004. PET measurements were available in 3702 [72%]. In these patients, high transporter status was found to be a significant, independent predictor of death-censored technique failure (adjusted hazard ratio [AHR] 1.23, 95% CI 1.02-1.49, p=0.03) and mortality (AHR 1.34, 95% CI 1.05-1.79, p=0.02) compared with low and low-average transporters. High-average transport status was also associated with mortality (AHR 1.21, 95% CI 1.00-1.48, p=0.047), but not death-censored technique failure (AHR 1.04, 95% CI 0.90-1.21).

6. Dialysis Adequacy According to Peritoneal Transport Status

6.1. Ultrafiltration

UF failure is an important clinical problem in patients on maintenance peritoneal dialysis. It may lead to severe fluid overload and subsequently congestive heart failure. The total incidence of impaired UF in PD is estimated to be between 10 and 40 percent [53]. The amount of UF is inversely proportional to the peritoneal transport of solutes, except in conditions of loss of surface area due to severe scarring/adhesions [54].

A diagnosis of UF failure is made when net UF < 100 ml after a 4-hour dwell with 2.5% glucose PD dialysate or < 400 ml with 4.25% glucose PD dialysate, in the absence of catheter malfunction, fluid leaks or extensive intraperitoneal adhesions [7, 55].

There are three types of UF failure:

- Type I membrane failure – associated with rapid solute transport
- Type II membrane failure – associated with impaired solute transport
- Type III membrane failure – associated with excessive lymphatic absorption

Type I membrane failure is the commonest type of UF failure. In this setting, equilibration across the membrane is so rapid that the osmotic gradient for glucose dissipates before adequate UF has had time to occur. Rapid transport status is present from the initiation of PD in minority of patients, whereas in others it appears with time. This UF loss is mainly associated with increased transport of low molecular weight solutes implying both a large effective peritoneal vascular surface area and impaired transcellular water transport [55].

High transporters on CAPD have consistently shown to have lower UF compared to other transport status. In the CANUSA study, the mean drain volumes in the PET for low, low-average, high-average and high transporters were 2.53 L, 2.45 L, 2.33 L and 2.16 L respectively. The consequence for high transporters is fluid retention and poor blood pressure control [40]. High transporter peritoneal membranes are prone to lose the osmotic gradient required for sustained ultrafiltration because of rapid absorption of glucose from the dialysate. As a consequence of this loss of osmotic gradient and subsequent decrease in ultrafiltration capacity, high transporters tend to have greater systemic exposure to glucose than low transporters do.

UF failure or inadequate UF is associated with high mortality and morbidity. UF failure, defined as a 24 hour peritoneal UF < 750 mL, was predictive of mortality in anuric automated peritoneal dialysis(APD) patients in the prospective observational European APD Outcome Study (EAPOS) [42]. Baseline UF rate, unlike creatinine clearance, was shown to be a significant predictor of survival by both univariate and multivariate analyses.

6.2. Solute Clearance

Inadequate solute clearance is defined as an increasing blood urea and plasma creatinine or the appearance of uraemic symptoms despite seemingly successful PD. There are different causes for inadequate solute clearance, including poor compliance, hypercatabolism and decreased peritoneal permeability. These various causes may be able to be distinguished by PET since peritoneal membrane transport status is one of the most important determinants of solute clearance. PD patients with low or low-average transport status have reduced solute clearance, whilst high and high-average transporters have increased solute clearance [56]. This helps to decide the best PD prescription for these patient groups

Badve and colleagues reported that the patients in the low-average and low membrane transport categories had lower peritoneal phosphate clearance than the high- average or the high membrane transport categories (33.2 + 8.5 versus 39.2 + 10.3 versus 49.6 + 11.4 L/wk/1.73 m2, respectively, $P < 0.001$) [57]. When peritoneal phosphate clearance by modality (CAPD Vs CCPD) was examined for each membrane category, there was no significant difference in phosphate clearance between the modalities in the high transport category. In the high-average category, however, there was significantly higher phosphate clearance among those treated with CAPD compared with CCPD (42.4 + 11.4 versus 36.4 + 8.3 L/wk/1.73 m2, $P = 0.01$). In the low-average and low membrane category, treatment with CAPD was associated with significantly higher phosphate clearance than CCPD (35.6 + 5.9 versus 28.9 + 11 L/wk/1.73 m2, $P = 0.034$). There was no significant difference in peritoneal creatinine clearance between the two modalities across any of the membrane transport categories.

7. Therapeutic Management

The management of these groups of patients can be challenging and involves various strategies.

7.1. Malnutrition and Hypoalbuminemia

Serum albumin is well known as a predictor of morbidity and mortality in PD patients [58]. Moreover, there appears to be an inverse correlation between D:P Cr and serum albumin [59].

In the CANUSA study, the mean serum albumin values for low, low-average, high-average and high transporters were 37.8 g/L, 36.2 g/L, 33.8 g/L and 32.8 g/L, respectively, and the mean peritoneal albumin losses were 3.1 g, 3.9 g, 4.3 g and 5.6 g, respectively [40]. Nolph and colleagues have also reported decreased lean body mass and lower normalized protein catabolic rate among high transporters over the long term [29]. It has been suggested that changing to APD might decrease these protein losses [59]. However, other studies have found protein losses to be similar in all types of PD therapies [60].

The nutritional status of PD patients should be closely monitored, particularly in high transporters. However, there is as yet no compelling evidence supporting any nutritional intervention. Oral calorie intake should be encouraged [61]. Intraperitoneal amino-acid solutions are commercially available but expensive. Moreover, the results of studies with intraperitoneal amino-acids have been conflicting. Kopple and colleagues showed some nutritional benefit with use of 1.1% amino-acid solution in malnourished CAPD patients [62]. However, most of these studies are underpowered and have short duration of follow up, thereby making it difficult to draw any firm conclusions about the clinical utility of this therapy.

7.2. Fluid Retention and Uncontrolled Blood Pressure

Inadequate UF is a common problem in high and high-average transporters. One of the methods to treat inadequate UF in high or high-average transporters is to shorten the dwell time of each exchange, thereby limiting the dialysis period to the time during which the osmotic gradient promoting UF is maximized. This is well achieved by automated PD. The cycler performs three to five short dwell exchanges during the sleeping period. Another approach would be to remove the excess fluid by utilizing hypertonic dextrose solutions. However, such solutions have been implicated in membrane damage and failure, and are associated with systemic side effects, such as hyperlipidaemia, obesity and glucose intolerance.

Icodextrin, a glucose polymer, may enhance UF in patients with high or high-average transport characteristics. Through colloid osmosis, it gives prolonged UF lasting 14-16 hours [63]. This mode of action implies that icodextrin is an appropriate agent for long dwells and not for short dwells. In the Midas multicenter trial, 7.5% icodextrin solution yielded better ultrafiltration than glucose solution even after 12 hours. Icodextrin use increases UF in a majority of patients, permitting reduction in the use of hypertonic dialysate. The consequent decrease in carbohydrate absorption should also lead to a better metabolic profile. Icodextrin is particularly indicated in patients with impaired ultrafiltration caused by a large peritoneal vascular surface area that leads to high transport of low molecular weight solute that is, high transporters. In a study of 33 patients with UF failure in which most were high and high-average transporters, the median increase in technique extension with the use of icodextrin was 22 months [64]. Another study comparing icodextrin with glucose dialysis solutions showed that icodextrin produced enhanced UF and clearances compared to 2.27% glucose, while avoiding exposure of the peritoneum to hypertonic glucose solution [65]. Icodextrin can possibly be used to enhance daytime UF during the long day dwell in patients on continuous cycling peritoneal dialysis (CCPD) who otherwise use glucose solution [81]. The same study showed higher 24-hour creatinine clearance in the group of patients that received icodextrin, possibly secondary to increased ultrafiltration.

7.3. Decreased Solute Clearances

Decreased small solute clearances are commonly observed in low and low-average transporters. The most efficient and least disruptive approach to increasing small solute clearance in low or low-average transporters is to increase dwell volume. Such a manoeuvre is usually well tolerated and leads to approximately a 20% increase in peritoneal clearance [66]. The alternative is to add a fifth exchange, which is less popular due to cost, noncompliance and lifestyle reasons [67, 68]. However, if this strategy is chosen, the most effective way to add the extra exchange would be to use a night exchange [69].

In APD patients, the most effective way to increase solute clearance is by adding a day time dwell in patients with ‘dry days’. The resulting increase in clearance is 30% to 35% [66]. If a day dwell is already being utilised, the addition of a second daytime exchange will also have a substantial effect, provided that each is in place for at least 4 hours to allow adequate solute equilibration.

Alternative methods to enhance clearance in APD patients are to increase the number of cycles per treatment session. However, this effect starts to plateau once the number of cycles exceeds about seven per 9-hour cycling session [66, 70]. Lengthening cycler time is also somewhat effective in increasing clearance, although at the cost of lifestyle constraints. Large dwell volumes, 4X2.5 L instead of 5X2 L, may give better clearance. However, the effect is modest and there are reports that higher volumes impair UF [71].

Juergensen and colleagues demonstrated that in high, high-average, and low-average transporters, clearances increased significantly when the dialysis volumes and number of exchanges were increased [72]. This is important as patients with large body mass lose renal function more rapidly. Moreover, adequate creatinine clearance can often not be attained in anuric patients, unless additional daytime exchanges are performed. The study included 11 patients on APD, of whom 6 were high or high-average transporters (group 1) and 5 were low transporters (group 2). For the group 1 patients, as total daily exchange volumes increased from 9.5 L to 14.5 L to 19.5 L, significant increases were observed in both Kpt/Vurea (1.68±0.21, 2.03 ± 0.28 and 2.28±0.28, respectively) and mean weekly creatinine clearance (45.43±7.63, 51.17±7.07 and 54.67±10.08 L/1.73 m^2). Similar findings were observed in the group 2 patients (mean weekly Kpt/Vurea 1.68±0.35, 2.10±0.42 and 2.31±0.56; mean weekly peritoneal creatinine clearance 42.56±10.64, 50.89±12.66 and 51.94 ± 11.20 L/1.73 m^2). Ultrafiltration was lower in the 9.5 L study than in the 14.5 L and 19.5-L studies, but was not different between the 14.5-L and 19.5-L studies.

Some authors have recommended APD instead of CAPD in high transporters to maximize both solute clearance and net UF as a result of the shorter dwell times achieved with APD [66]. In a retrospective study of PD patients in Taiwan, high transporters had a lower probability of survival on APD over a mean of two years, although technique survival was not decreased. However, in this study only 5 patients (10% of the total) were high transporters, and these patients were using different APD prescriptions from patients of other transport types [23]. Moreover, there was no direct comparison of APD versus CAPD treatment in this population. A subsequent ANZDATA Registry investigation by our group demonstrated that APD treatment was associated with a significant overall survival advantage in high transporters compared with CAPD, although death-censored technique survival was comparable between the two modalities. On the other hand, APD treatment is associated with inferior survival in low transporters [73]. In this study out of the 4128 PD patients 628 were high transporters (486 on CAPD and 142 on APD). On multivariate intention- to-treat analysis, APD treatment was associated with superior survival [adjusted hazard ratio [74] 0.56, 95% confidence interval [75] 0.35–0.87) and comparable death-censored technique survival (HR 0.88, 95% CI 0.64–1.21). Superior survival of high transporters treated with APD versus CAPD was also confirmed in supplemental as-treated analysis (HR 0.72, 95% CI 0.54–0.96), matched case-control analysis (HR 0.60, 95% CI 0.36–0.96) and subgroup analysis of high transporters treated entirely with APD versus those treated entirely with CAPD (HR 0.29, 95% CI 0.14–0.60). There were no statistically significant differences in patient survival or death-censored technique survival between APD and CAPD for any other transport group, except for low transporters, who experienced a higher mortality rate on APD compared with CAPD (HR 2.19, 95% CI 1.02–4.70). The reasons for this observation are not known, but possibly relate to reduced small solute clearances in low transports on APD due to repeated drain-fill cycles leading to reduced membrane contact time).

Summary

Peritoneal transport status is a key characteristic of the peritoneal membrane that is strongly associated with peritoneal UF, small solute clearance, nutrition and survival. Although peritoneal transport can be measured via a variety of methods, the most common technique involves measurement of the ratio of dialysate to plasma concentration of creatinine following a 4 hour dwell of 2 L of 2.5% glucose dialysate (D:P Cr) using a Peritoneal Equilibration Test (PET). Transport status is typically categorised into 4 groups according to the mean ± 1 standard deviation of D:P Cr: High (D:P Cr ≥0.81, 16%), High-average (D:P Cr 0.65-0.80, 51%), Low-average (D:P Cr 0.50-0.64, 28%), and Low (D:P Cr <0.50, 5%). High transporters on chronic PD are challenged by increased protein losses, high glucose absorption, and poor UF and are best treated with short dwell APD regimens overnight in concert with daytime icodextrin exchanges. On the other hand, low transporters are challenged by diminished small solute clearance and are optimally treated by long dwell CAPD regimens to achieve improved survival outcomes. Consequently, determination of an individual's peritoneal transport status represents an important risk-stratification tool to guide PD therapy and optimise clinical outcomes.

FUTURE RESEARCH DIRECTIONS

Currently available tests for peritoneal membrane transport status are focused on small solute clearances. These tests require frequent sampling, and thus are labour- and time-consuming. Further studies are required to develop new tests that are accurate and easy to perform and interpret. Assessment of peritoneal membrane transport status should not only relate to small solute clearances, but also middle molecule clearance, ultrafiltration capacity with different PD solutions, and metabolic consequences. Future studies should focus on important and poorly understood issues such as intra-patient variability, reproducibility, and optimal frequency of tests that is clinically meaningful. Future research should be centred around patient-related issues, such as derivation of peritoneal membrane transport status-based therapies and clinical outcomes.

REFERENCES

[1] Margetts PJ, Brimble KS. Peritoneal dialysis, membranes and beyond. Curr Opin Nephrol Hypertens. [Research Support, Non-U.S. Gov't Review]. 2006 Nov;15(6):571-6.

[2] Chung SH, Heimburger O, Lindholm B, Lee HB. Peritoneal dialysis patient survival: a comparison between a Swedish and a Korean centre. Nephrol Dial Transplant. [Comparative Study Multicenter Study]. 2005 Jun;20(6):1207-13.

[3] Churchill DN, Thorpe KE, Nolph KD, Keshaviah PR, Oreopoulos DG, Page D. Increased peritoneal membrane transport is associated with decreased patient and technique survival for continuous peritoneal dialysis patients. The Canada-USA (CANUSA) Peritoneal Dialysis Study Group. J Am Soc Nephrol. [Clinical Trial Multicenter Study Research Support, Non-U.S. Gov't]. 1998 Jul;9(7):1285-92.

[4] Davies SJ, Phillips L, Naish PF, Russell GI. Quantifying comorbidity in peritoneal dialysis patients and its relationship to other predictors of survival. Nephrol Dial Transplant. [Research Support, Non-U.S. Gov't]. 2002 Jun;17(6):1085-92.

[5] Fried L. Higher membrane permeability predicts poorer patient survival. Perit Dial Int. 1997 Jul-Aug;17(4):387-9.

[6] Wang T, Heimburger O, Waniewski J, Bergstrom J, Lindholm B. Increased peritoneal permeability is associated with decreased fluid and small-solute removal and higher mortality in CAPD patients. Nephrol Dial Transplant. [Research Support, Non-U.S. Gov't]. 1998 May;13(5):1242-9.

[7] Twardowski Z, Nolph KD, Khanna R. Peritoneal equilibration test. Perit Dial Bull. 1987;7:138-47.

[8] Johnson DW, Mudge DW, Blizzard S, Arndt M, O'Shea A, Watt R, et al. A comparison of peritoneal equilibration tests performed 1 and 4 weeks after PD commencement. Perit Dial Int. 2004 Sep-Oct;24(5):460-5.

[9] Haraldsson B. Assessing the peritoneal dialysis capacities of individual patients. Kidney Int. 1995 Apr;47(4):1187-98.

[10] La Milia V, Di Filippo S, Crepaldi M, Del Vecchio L, Dell'Oro C, Andrulli S, et al. Mini-peritoneal equilibration test: A simple and fast method to assess free water and small solute transport across the peritoneal membrane. Kidney Int. [Clinical Trial Comparative Study]. 2005 Aug;68(2):840-6.

[11] La Milia V, Limardo M, Virga G, Crepaldi M, Locatelli F. Simultaneous measurement of peritoneal glucose and free water osmotic conductances. Kidney Int. [Clinical Trial]. 2007 Sep;72(5):643-50.

[12] Van Biesen W, Van der Tol A, Veys N, Dequidt C, Vijt D, Lameire N, et al. The personal dialysis capacity test is superior to the peritoneal equilibration test to discriminate inflammation as the cause of fast transport status in peritoneal dialysis patients. Clin J Am Soc Nephrol. 2006 Mar;1(2):269-74.

[13] Prowant BF, Moore HL, Twardowski ZJ, Khanna R. Understanding discrepancies in peritoneal equilibration test results. Perit Dial Int. 2010 May-Jun;30(3):366-70.

[14] Voinescu CG, Khanna R, Nolph KD. High peritoneal transport: a blessing or curse? Adv Perit Dial. 2002;18:106-11.

[15] Correa-Rotter R, Cueto-Manzano A. The problem of the high transporter: is survival decreased? Perit Dial Int. 2001;21 Suppl 3:S75-9.

[16] Rumpsfeld M, McDonald SP, Johnson DW. Higher peritoneal transport status is associated with higher mortality and technique failure in the Australian and New Zealand peritoneal dialysis patient populations. J Am Soc Nephrol. 2006 Jan;17(1):271-8.

[17] Raj DS, Langos V, Gangam N, Roscoe J. Ethnic variability in peritoneal equilibration test and urea kinetics. Am J Kidney Dis. 1997 Sep; 30(3):374-81.

[18] Cueto-Manzano AM, Diaz-Alvarenga A, Correa-Rotter R. Analysis of the peritoneal equilibration test in Mexico and factors influencing the peritoneal transport rate. Perit Dial Int. 1999 Jan-Feb;19(1):45-50.
[19] Passadakis PS, Thodis ED, Panagoutsos SA, Selisiou CA, Pitta EM, Vargemezis VA. Outcome for continuous ambulatory peritoneal dialysis patients is not predicted by peritoneal permeability characteristics. Adv Perit Dial. 2000;16:2-6.
[20] Agrawal A, Nolph KD. Management of high peritoneal transporters. Perit Dial Int. [Review]. 2000;20 Suppl 2:S160-5.
[21] Cueto-Manzano AM, Correa-Rotter R. Is high peritoneal transport rate an independent risk factor for CAPD mortality? Kidney Int. 2000;57(1):314-20.
[22] Wu CH, Huang CC, Huang JY, Wu MS, Leu ML. High flux peritoneal membrane is a risk factor in survival of CAPD treatment. Adv Perit Dial. 1996;12:105-9.
[23] Hung KY, Lin TJ, Tsai TJ, Chen WY. Impact of peritoneal membrane transport on technique failure and patient survival in a population on automated peritoneal dialysis. Asaio J. 1999 Nov-Dec;45(6):568-73.
[24] Park MS, Lee HA, Chu WS, Yang DH, Hwang SD. Peritoneal accumulation of AGE and peritoneal membrane permeability. Perit Dial Int. 2000 Jul-Aug;20(4):452-60.
[25] Schwedler S, Schinzel R, Vaith P, Wanner C. Inflammation and advanced glycation end products in uremia: simple coexistence, potentiation or causal relationship? Kidney Int Suppl. 2001 Feb;78:S32-6.
[26] Teillet L, Verbeke P, Gouraud S, Bakala H, Borot-Laloi C, Heudes D, et al. Food restriction prevents advanced glycation end product accumulation and retards kidney aging in lean rats. J Am Soc Nephrol. 2000 Aug;11(8):1488-97.
[27] Bergstrom J, Lindholm B. Malnutrition, cardiac disease, and mortality: an integrated point of view. Am J Kidney Dis. 1998 Nov;32(5):834-41.
[28] Cueto-Manzano AM, Gamba G, Correa-Rotter R. Peritoneal protein loss in patients with high peritoneal permeability: comparison between continuous ambulatory peritoneal dialysis and daytime intermittent peritoneal dialysis. Arch Med Res. 2001 May-Jun;32(3):197-201.
[29] Nolph KD, Moore HL, Prowant B, Twardowski ZJ, Khanna R, Gamboa S, et al. Continuous ambulatory peritoneal dialysis with a high flux membrane. Asaio J. 1993 Oct-Dec;39(4):904-9.

[30] Szeto CC, Law MC, Wong TY, Leung CB, Li PK. Peritoneal transport status correlates with morbidity but not longitudinal change of nutritional status of continuous ambulatory peritoneal dialysis patients: a 2-year prospective study. Am J Kidney Dis. 2001 Feb;37(2):329-36.
[31] Cueto-Manzano AM, Espinosa A, Hernandez A, Correa-Rotter R. Peritoneal transport kinetics correlate with serum albumin but not with the overall nutritional status in CAPD patients. Am J Kidney Dis. 1997 Aug;30(2):229-36.
[32] Breborowicz A, Oreopoulos DG. Evidence for the presence of chronic inflammation during peritoneal dialysis: therapeutic implications. Perit Dial Int. 1997;17 Suppl 2:S37-41.
[33] Chung SH, Heimburger O, Stenvinkel P, Qureshi AR, Lindholm B. Association between residual renal function, inflammation and patient survival in new peritoneal dialysis patients. Nephrol Dial Transplant. 2003 Mar;18(3):590-7.
[34] Wang T, Heimburger O, Cheng HH, Bergstrom J, Lindholm B. Does a high peritoneal transport rate reflect a state of chronic inflammation? Perit Dial Int. 1999 Jan-Feb;19(1):17-22.
[35] Herzig KA, Purdie DM, Chang W, Brown AM, Hawley CM, Campbell SB, et al. Is C-reactive protein a useful predictor of outcome in peritoneal dialysis patients? J Am Soc Nephrol. 2001 Apr;12(4):814-21.
[36] Kennedy R, Case C, Fathi R, Johnson D, Isbel N, Marwick TH. Does renal failure cause an atherosclerotic milieu in patients with end-stage renal disease? Am J Med. 2001 Feb 15;110(3):198-204.
[37] Williams JD, Craig KJ, Topley N, Von Ruhland C, Fallon M, Newman GR, et al. Morphologic changes in the peritoneal membrane of patients with renal disease. J Am Soc Nephrol. 2002 Feb;13(2):470-9.
[38] Wilmer WA, Pesavento TE, Bay WH, Middendorf DF, Donelan SE, Frabott SM, et al. Peritoneal dialysis following failed kidney transplantation is associated with high peritoneal transport rates. Perit Dial Int. 2001 Jul-Aug;21(4):411-3.
[39] Heimburger O, Waniewski J, Werynski A, Tranaeus A, Lindholm B. Peritoneal transport in CAPD patients with permanent loss of ultrafiltration capacity. Kidney Int. [Comparative Study Research Support, Non-U.S. Gov't]. 1990 Sep;38(3):495-506.
[40] Churchill DN, Thorpe KE, Nolph KD, Keshaviah PR, Oreopoulos DG, Page D. for the Canada-USA (CANUSA) Peritoneal Dialysis Study Group: Increased peritoneal membrane transport is associated with

decreased patient and technique survival for continuous peritoneal dialysis patients. J Am Soc Nephrol. 1998;9:1285-92.
[41] Davies SJ, Phillips L, Russell GI. Peritoneal solute transport predicts survival on CAPD independently of residual renal function. Nephrol Dial Transplant. [Research Support, Non-U.S. Gov't]. 1998 Apr;13(4):962-8.
[42] Brown EA, Davies SJ, Rutherford P, Meeus F, Borras M, Riegel W, et al. Survival of functionally anuric patients on automated peritoneal dialysis: the European APD Outcome Study. J Am Soc Nephrol. 2003 Nov;14(11):2948-57.
[43] Paniagua R, Amato D, Vonesh E, Correa-Rotter R, Ramos A, Moran J, et al. Effects of increased peritoneal clearances on mortality rates in peritoneal dialysis: ADEMEX, a prospective, randomized, controlled trial. J Am Soc Nephrol. 2002 May;13(5):1307-20.
[44] Park HC, Kang SW, Choi KH, Ha SK, Han DS, Lee HY. Clinical outcome in continuous ambulatory peritoneal dialysis patients is not influenced by high peritoneal transport status. Perit Dial Int. 2001;21 Suppl 3:S80-5.
[45] Chung SH, Heimburger O, Stenvinkel P, Wang T, Lindholm B. Influence of peritoneal transport rate, inflammation, and fluid removal on nutritional status and clinical outcome in prevalent peritoneal dialysis patients. Perit Dial Int. 2003 Mar-Apr;23(2):174-83.
[46] Ates K, Nergizoglu G, Keven K, Sen A, Kutlay S, Erturk S, et al. Effect of fluid and sodium removal on mortality in peritoneal dialysis patients. Kidney Int. 2001 Aug;60(2):767-76.
[47] Blake PG. What is the problem with high transporters? Perit Dial Int. 1997 Jul-Aug;17(4):317-20.
[48] Tzamaloukas AH, Saddler MC, Murata GH, Malhotra D, Sena P, Simon D, et al. Symptomatic fluid retention in patients on continuous peritoneal dialysis. J Am Soc Nephrol. 1995 Aug;6(2):198-206.
[49] Chung SH, Chu WS, Lee HA, Kim YH, Lee IS, Lindholm B, et al. Peritoneal transport characteristics, comorbid diseases and survival in CAPD patients. Perit Dial Int. 2000 Sep-Oct;20(5):541-7.
[50] Han DS, Lee SW, Kang SW, Choi KH, Lee HY, Cho EY, et al. Factors affecting low values of serum albumin in CAPD patients. Adv Perit Dial. 1996;12:288-92.
[51] Fung L, Pollock CA, Caterson RJ, Mahony JF, Waugh DA, Macadam C, et al. Dialysis adequacy and nutrition determine prognosis in continuous

ambulatory peritoneal dialysis patients. J Am Soc Nephrol. 1996 May;7(5):737-44.
[52] Struijk DG, Krediet RT, Koomen GC, Boeschoten EW, Hoek FJ, Arisz L. A prospective study of peritoneal transport in CAPD patients. Kidney Int. 1994 Jun;45(6):1739-44.
[53] Smit W, Schouten N, van den Berg N, Langedijk MJ, Struijk DG, Krediet RT. Analysis of the prevalence and causes of ultrafiltration failure during long-term peritoneal dialysis: a cross-sectional study. Perit Dial Int. 2004 Nov-Dec;24(6):562-70.
[54] Pollock CA, Ibels LS, Hallett MD, Cocksedge B, Caterson RJ, Mahony JF, et al. Loss of ultrafiltration in continuous ambulatory peritoneal dialysis (CAPD). Perit Dial Int. 1989;9(2):107-10.
[55] Ho-dac-Pannekeet MM, Atasever B, Struijk DG, Krediet RT. Analysis of ultrafiltration failure in peritoneal dialysis patients by means of standard peritoneal permeability analysis. Perit Dial Int. 1997 Mar-Apr;17(2):144-50.
[56] Twardowski ZJ, Nolph KD, Khanna R, Prowant BF, Ryan LP, Moore HL, et al. Peritoneal equilibration test. Perit Dial Bull. 1987;7:138-47.
[57] Badve SV, Zimmerman DL, Knoll GA, Burns KD, McCormick BB. Peritoneal phosphate clearance is influenced by peritoneal dialysis modality, independent of peritoneal transport characteristics. Clinical journal of the American Society of Nephrology : CJASN. [Comparative Study]. 2008 Nov;3(6):1711-7.
[58] Blake PG, Flowerdew G, Blake RM, Oreopoulos DG. Serum albumin in patients on continuous ambulatory peritoneal dialysis--predictors and correlations with outcomes. J Am Soc Nephrol. 1993 Feb;3(8):1501-7.
[59] Burkart JM. Effect of peritoneal dialysis prescription and peritoneal membrane transport characteristics on nutritional status. Perit Dial Int. [Review]. 1995;15(5 Suppl):S20-35.
[60] Kathuria P, Moore HL, Khanna R, Twardowski ZJ, Goel S, Nolph KD. Effect of dialysis modality and membrane transport characteristics on dialysate protein losses of patients on peritoneal dialysis. Perit Dial Int. 1997 Sep-Oct;17(5):449-54.
[61] Donate T OA, Facundo C, Martinez, Roda M, Barcelo P. Oral protein supplement efficacy in peritoneal dialysis patients. Perit Dial Int. 1999;19(Suppl 1):S15.
[62] Kopple JD, Bernard D, Messana J, Swartz R, Bergstrom J, Lindholm B, et al. Treatment of malnourished CAPD patients with an amino acid

based dialysate. Kidney Int. [Clinical Trial Multicenter Study]. 1995 Apr;47(4):1148-57.

[63] Mistry CD, Gokal R, Peers E. A randomized multicenter clinical trial comparing isosmolar icodextrin with hyperosmolar glucose solutions in CAPD. MIDAS Study Group. Multicenter Investigation of Icodextrin in Ambulatory Peritoneal Dialysis. Kidney Int. 1994 Aug;46(2):496-503.

[64] Wilkie ME, Plant MJ, Edwards L, Brown CB. Icodextrin 7.5% dialysate solution (glucose polymer) in patients with ultrafiltration failure: extension of CAPD technique survival. Perit Dial Int. 1997 Jan-Feb;17(1):84-7.

[65] Woodrow G, Stables G, Oldroyd B, Gibson J, Turney JH, Brownjohn AM. Comparison of icodextrin and glucose solutions for the daytime dwell in automated peritoneal dialysis. Nephrol Dial Transplant. [Comparative Study Research Support, Non-U.S. Gov't]. 1999 Jun;14(6):1530-5.

[66] Blake P, Burkart JM, Churchill DN, Daugirdas J, Depner T, Hamburger RJ, et al. Recommended clinical practices for maximizing peritoneal dialysis clearances. Perit Dial Int. 1996 Sep-Oct;16(5):448-56.

[67] Blake PG, Floyd J, Spanner E, Peters K. How much extra does "adequate" peritoneal dialysis cost? Perit Dial Int. [Research Support, Non-U.S. Gov't]. 1996; 16 Suppl 1:S171-5.

[68] Blake PG, Korbet SM, Blake R, Bargman JM, Burkart JM, Delano BG, et al. A multicenter study of noncompliance with continuous ambulatory peritoneal dialysis exchanges in US and Canadian patients. Am J Kidney Dis. [Comparative Study Multicenter Study Research Support, Non-U.S. Gov't]. 2000 Mar;35(3):506-14.

[69] Page DE. CAPD with a night-exchange device is the only true CAPD? Adv Perit Dial. [Comparative Study]. 1998;14:60-3.

[70] Perez RA, Blake PG, McMurray S, Mupas L, Oreopoulos DG. What is the optimal frequency of cycling in automated peritoneal dialysis? Perit Dial Int. [Clinical Trial Comparative Study Research Support, Non-U.S. Gov't]. 2000 Sep-Oct;20(5):548-56.

[71] Durand PY, Balteau P, Chanliau J. Dwell volume prescription in automated peritoneal dialysis and its assessment. Contrib Nephrol. [Review]. 1999;129:90-7.

[72] Juergensen PH, Murphy AL, Kliger AS, Finkelstein FO. Increasing the dialysis volume and frequency in a fixed period of time in CPD patients: the effect on Kpt/V and creatinine clearance. Perit Dial Int. [Clinical Trial]. 2002 Nov-Dec;22(6):693-7.

[73] Johnson DW, Hawley CM, McDonald SP, Brown FG, Rosman JB, Wiggins KJ, et al. Superior survival of high transporters treated with automated versus continuous ambulatory peritoneal dialysis. Nephrol Dial Transplant. [Comparative Study]. 2010 Jun;25(6):1973-9.

[74] Finkelstein F, Healy H, Abu-Alfa A, Ahmad S, Brown F, Gehr T, et al. Superiority of icodextrin compared with 4.25% dextrose for peritoneal ultrafiltration. J Am Soc Nephrol. 2005 Feb;16(2):546-54.

[75] Selgas R, Bajo MA, Castro MJ, Sanchez-Tomero JA, Cirugeda A. Managing ultrafiltration failure by peritoneal resting. Perit Dial Int. 2000 Nov-Dec;20(6):595-7.

In: Peritoneal Dialysis
Editors: A. Agarwal, L. Salman et al.
ISBN: 978-1-62257-896-2

Chapter 4

INFECTION AND PERITONEAL DIALYSIS

Nabil J. Haddad

ABSTRACT

Peritoneal dialysis related infections are a major cause of morbidity and mortality in patients with end-stage kidney disease undergoing peritoneal dialysis. Prevention, early recognition and adequate management of these infections are of paramount importance. Exit site, tunnel infections and CAPD-associated peritonitis need to be differentiated and aggressively treated, and may result in the loss of this option of renal replacement therapy. The knowledge of different etiologic factors, signs and symptoms and adequate therapy of each entity of PD-related infection markedly improve the outcomes in these patients.

INTRODUCTION

Infection is a major complication of peritoneal dialysis and may result in loss of this option of renal replacement therapy [1, 2]. Peritoneal dialysis related infections include both exit site and tunnel infections, in addition to peritonitis. The different kinds of PD infections increase both morbidity and mortality in dialysis maintained patients, related to each other and may coexist in a single patient. The following chapter will cover definition, etiology, diagnosis and management of each entity.

Exit Site Infection

Definition: The presence of purulent discharge from the exit site, with or without surrounding erythema [3, 4]. It is usually located in the catheter-skin interface and does not extend beyond the external PD catheter cuff.

Etiology: Exit site infection is usually caused by bacteria colonizing the catheter and skin [5]. It is caused by different micro-organisms but Staphylococcus aureus, Staphylococcus epidermidis and Pseudomonas aeruginosa account for the majority of exit site infections. Usually bacteria colonize the PD catheter soon after placement and may form a biofilm, which forms a barrier against antimicrobials and facilitates its growth. This later may lead to subsequent tissue infiltration and infection.

Diagnosis: The major sign of exit site infection is purulent discharge at the catheter-skin junction. Soreness and pericatheter erythema may also be present [4, 6]. Positive cultures from the exit site confirm the diagnosis and direct the choice of antibiotic therapy.

Management: Both aerobic and anaerobic cultures and gram stain of exit site should be obtained, with the caveat that positive cultures in the absence of purulent discharge may result from colonization. The presence of pericatheter erythema without discharge may be treated with topical antimicrobials (diluted hydrogen peroxide and chlorhexidine) twice daily and without the use of occlusive dressing. If discharge is present, empiric oral antibiotic therapy covering Staphylococcus (penicillinase-resistant or first generation cephalosporin) should be utilized [7]. Gram-negative infections require therapy with fluoroquinolones. The antibiotic therapy should be continued until normalization of the exit site appearance and for at least two weeks duration [3]. The choice of antibiotics should be adjusted after the results of gram stain and culture. PD catheter removal is indicated in the presence of fungal and resistant (more that 3 weeks of appropriate antibiotic therapy] infections, or co-existence of a tunnel infection. Prophylaxis with topical antimicrobials and exit site care is recommended [8].

Tunnel Infection

Definition: The presence of erythema, edema and tenderness over the PD catheter subcutaneous tunnel [3] it is localized to catheter length between the two cuffs.

Etiology: As in exit site infection it can result from a variety of micro-organisms and most commonly by Staphylococcus and Pseudomonas species.

Diagnosis: Tenderness over the subcutaneous tunnel of PD catheter that is associated with erythema and edema is the whole mark of tunnel infection. It is frequently associated with exit site infection and may have no apparent clinical symptoms [9]. Ultrasound evaluation may confirm the diagnosis of tunnel site infection [10].

Management: PD catheter removal with perioperative antibiotic therapy is the treatment of choice [4]. The antibiotic therapy needs to be continued for at least 10 days after removal of the PD catheter.

Peritonitis in Peritoneal Dialysis

Definition: Inflammation of the peritoneum related to infectious etiology in patients maintained on peritoneal dialysis.

Etiology: Bacterial pathogens are the most common etiologic culprits in PD peritonitis, while other cases may be caused by fungi, especially Candida species. The presence of viral peritonitis is uncertain. Coagulase negative and coagulase-positive Staphylococci account for about 50% PD peritonitis and usually result from touch contamination or exit site and tunnel infections. Gram-negative micro-organisms account for 15-20% of PD peritonitis, while the rest is caused by polymicrobial flora and fungi, or may be culture negative in up to 20% of cases.

Diagnosis: Peritonitis should always be considered in any patient on PD, who presents with abdominal pain and cloudy peritoneal fluid. Other symptoms and signs may include fever, nausea, diarrhea and abdominal tenderness with or without rebound [11].

The diagnosis can be confirmed by the following findings:

1. PD fluid WBC count of more than 100 per mm3 with ≥ 50% Europhiles after at least 2 hours of dwell time.
2. Positive gram stain and fluid culture.
3. Broad spectrum PCR with RNA sequencing and quantitative bacterial DNA PCR may also assist in diagnosis.

It is of paramount importance to differentiate between peritonitis secondary to touch contamination and catheter-related infection, and secondary peritonitis related to underlying gastrointestinal etiology, which includes bowel perforation, appendicitis, cholecystitis, bowel ischemia, incarcerated hernia and other etiologies. The presence of polymicrobial bacteria and high amylase level (above 50 IU/L) in the PD fluid is suggestive of a secondary etiology. Abdominal CT scan, magnetic resonance imaging and radionuclide scanning are very helpful in these cases to rule out a secondary etiology.

Management: Empiric antibiotic therapy covering both Gram positive and Gram negative is recommended [6]. Intraperitoneal antibiotic therapy is the preferred route of antibiotic administration [3]. The combination of Vancomycin or a cephalosporin to cover Gram positive micro-organisms and an aminoglycoside or a third generation cephalosporin to cover Gram negative bacteria is the widely accepted regimen of antimicrobial therapy. The choice of antibiotics should be adjusted after obtaining the results of PD fluid culture (tables 2 and 3]. Either continuous or intermittent administration of antibiotics is effective and needs to be followed by drug level for appropriate dosing. The duration of therapy depends on the causative organisms with the least duration of 2 weeks of antibiotic administration. PD peritonitis secondary to Pseudomonas aeruginosa should be treated with two antibiotics and for duration of 3 weeks. Stenotrophomonas related peritonitis should also be treated with 2 antibiotics and for duration of 3-4 weeks.

In patients with **culture negative peritonitis**, if repeat PD fluid cell count and symptoms improve within 3-4 days, empiric therapy is usually continued for 2 weeks. Otherwise, it is recommended to obtain cultures for uncommon etiologic organisms like fungi, mycobacterium and mycoplasma [4].

Refractory peritonitis is defined as PD peritonitis that fails to respond to appropriate antibiotic therapy after 5 days while relapsing peritonitis is the term used for peritonitis that recurs within 4 weeks of completion of therapy with the same pathogen or one sterile episode. Recurrent peritonitis is defined as another episode that occurs within 4 weeks after completing therapy with a different pathogen and repeat peritonitis is an episode that occurs more the 4 weeks after completing antibiotic course with the same micro-organism. The removal of PD catheter may be indicated in some cases (table 1; Ref: [4, 6].

Table 1. Indications for PD catheter removal

1. Refractory peritonitis.
2. Relapsing peritonitis.
3. Fungal peritonitis.
4. Peritonitis associated with tunnel infection or resistant exit site infection.

Table 2. Intraperitoneal Antibiotic Dosing Recommendations for CAPD Patients (Printed by permission of ISPD)

	Intermittent Dosing (per exchange once daily)	Continuous (mg/L; all exchanges
Aminoglycosides		
Amikacin	2 mg/kg	LD 25, MD 12
Gent, tobro, netlimicin	0.6 mg/kg	LD 8, MD 4
Cephalosporins		
Cefazolin,cephalothin,cephradine	15 mg/kg	LD 500, MD 125
Cefepime	1000 mg	LD 500, MD 125
Ceftazidime	1000- 1500 mg	LD 500, MD 125
Ceftizoxime	1000 mg	LD 250, MD 125
Penicillins		
Amoxicillin	ND	LD 250–500, MD 50
Ampicillin, oxacillin, or nafcillin	ND	MD 125
Azlocillin	ND	LD 500, MD 250
Penicillin G (units)	ND	LD 50000 , MD 25000
Quinolones		
Ciprofloxacin	ND	LD 50, MD 25
Others		
Aztreonam	ND	LD 1000, MD 250
Daptomycin	ND	LD 100, MD 20
Linezolid (Oral 200–300 mg q.d)		
Teicoplanin	15 mg/kg	LD 400, MD 20
Vancomycin	15–30 mg/kg every 5–7	LD 1000, MD 25

Table 2.(Continued)

	Intermittent Dosing (per exchange once daily)	Continuous (mg/L; all exchanges
Antifungals		
Amphotericin	NA	1.5
Fluconazole	200 mg IP every 24–48 hours	
Combinations		
Ampicillin/sulbactam	2 g every 12 hours	LD 1000, MD 100
Imipenem/cilastin	1 g b.i.d.	LD 250, MD 50
Quinupristin/dalfopristin	25 mg/L in alternate bags (b)	
Trimethoprim/sulfamethoxazole Oral 960 mg b.i.d.		

ND = no data; q.d. = every day; NA = not applicable; IP = intraperitoneal; b.i.d. = 2 times per day; LD = loading dose in mg/L; MD = maintenance dose in mg/L. (a) For dosing of drugs with renal clearance in patients with residual renal function (defined as >100 mL/day urine output), dose should be empirically increased by 25%. (b) Given in conjunction with 500 mg intravenous twice daily.

Table 3. Intermittent Dosing of Antibiotics in Automated Peritoneal Dialysis (Printed by permission of ISPD)

Drug	**IP dose**
Cefazolin	20 mg/kg IP every day, in long day dwell
Cefepime	1 g IP in 1 exchange per day
Fluconazole	200 mg IP in 1 exchange per day every 24–48 hours
Tobramycin	LD 1.5 mg/kg IP in long dwell, then 0.5 mg/kg IP each day in long dwell
Vancomycin	LD 30 mg/kg IP in long dwell; repeat dosing 15 mg/kg IP in long dwell every 3–5 days (aim to keep serum trough levels above 15 μg/mL)

IP = intraperitoneal; LD = loading dose.

REFERENCES

[1] Guo, A, Mujais, S. Patient and technique survival for patients on PD in the US: Evaluation in large incident cohorts. Kidney Int 2003; 64:S3-S12.

[2] Stablein DM, Nolph KD, Lindblad AS. Timing and characteristics of multiple peritonitis.

[3] ISPD guildelines/recommendations. Peritoneal Dialysis International, Vol. 30, p 393-423. 2010, accessed June 2011.

[4] Piraino B, Bailie GR, Bernardini J, Boeschoten E, Gupta A, Holmes C, Kuijper EJ, Li PK, Lye WC, Mujais S, Paterson DL, Fontan MP, Ramos A, Schaefer F, Uttley L. Peritoneal dialysis-related infections recommendations: 2005 update. Peritoneal Dialysis Int. 2005; 25:107-31

[5] A Scalamongna, C Castelnovo, A De Vecchi, C Penticelli. Exit site and tunnel infections in continuous ambulatory peritoneal dialysis patients. AJKD 1991; 18:674.

[6] LI PK, Szeto CC. Paraino B, et al. Peritoneal Dialysis-related Infections recommendations. 2010 update. Perit Dial Int 2010; 30:393.

[7] Twardowski ZJ, Prowant BF. Current approach to exit-site infections in patients on peritoneal dialysis. Nephrology Dial Transplant 1997; 12:1284.

[8] Pirano B, Bernardini J, Bender FH. An analysis of methods to prevent peritoneal dialysis catheter infections. Perit Dial Int 2008; 28:437.

[9] Plum J, Sudkamp S, Grabensee B. Results of ultra sound assisted diagnosis of tunnel infections in continuous ambulatory peritoneal dialysis. Am J Kidney Dis 1994; 23:99-104.

[10] Kwan TH, Tong MK, Siu YP, Leung KT, Luk SH, Cheung YK. Utrasonography in the management of exit site infections in peritoneal dialysis patients. Nephrology (Carlton) 2004: 9:348.

[11] Vas, SI. Peritonitis. In: Peritoneal Dialysis, 3rd ed, Nolph, KD (Eds), Kluwer Academic Publishers, Dordrecht 1989. p.261.

In: Peritoneal Dialysis
Editors: A. Agarwal, L. Salman et al.
ISBN: 978-1-62257-896-2

Chapter 5

PERITONEAL DIALYSIS IN CONGESTIVE HEART FAILURE: A CONTEMPORARY, EVIDENCE-BASED REVIEW

***Amit Kaushal*[1], *Shelley Zieroth*[1,2], *Martina Reslerova*[1,2], *Mauro Verrelli*[1,2], *Paul Komenda*[1,3], *Claudio Rigatto*[1, 3] and *Manish M. Sood*[1,2*]**

[1] University of Manitoba, Winnipeg, Manitoba, Canada
[2] St Boniface Hospital, Winnipeg, Manitoba, Canada
[3] Seven Oaks Hospital, Winnipeg, Manitoba, Canada

ABSTRACT

A fundamental role of dialysis in the end stage renal disease (ESRD) population is optimizing extracellular fluid management in the context of abnormal autoregulation. This problem is shared with many other medical conditions such as congestive heart failure (CHF). Peritoneal dialysis, with its slow, continuous ultrafiltration, has been utilized in CHF in patients with and without other indications for kidney replacement therapy. The evidence supporting such an approach in this "non-ESRD" population is limited, and predominantly founded on case series and observational studies. In this review, we will examine the role of PD in

* Corresponding Author. Tel: 204-237-2121, FAX: 204-233-2770

the CHF population. Namely we will review the existing literature outlining the populations studied and their outcomes both PD-related (peritonitis, technique failure) and non-PD-related (mortality, hospitalizations, quality of life).

INTRODUCTION

The optimal management of congestive heart failure (CHF) is a problem of growing significance in everyday practice. Evidence based therapies for CHF have been effective in reducing mortality and hospitalizations while improving quality of life [1-4]. Unfortunately, despite the use of diuretics, blockade of the renin-angiotensin axis and further pharmacologic measures to improve both preload and afterload, there remains a cohort of patients with refractory disease often requiring therapies such as intravenous diuretics, supplemental oxygen. These patients commonly suffer from limitations in functional capacity as defined by New York Heart Association (NYHA) class, are plagued by fluid overload as well as hyponatremia (another negative prognosticator of mortality) [5-7], and poor quality of life. Many patients with CHF are also known to have chronic kidney disease (CKD), with cardiovascular disease being the most common cause of death in this population [8, 9]. In a large database of 105,388 patients compiled by the Acute Decompensated Heart Failure National Registry requiring, 30% had concomitant CKD, varying from stage 1 to stage 5 as defined by National Kidney Foundation Kidney Disease Outcomes Quality Initiative [10]. The majority of these patients had stage III disease; in 20% and 9% of patients, serum creatinine was greater than 176 μmol/L and 264 μmol/L, respectively, and another 5% were receiving dialysis therapy. Additionally, in a 2004 prospective study of 6,427 patients with a clinical diagnosis of CHF and coronary artery disease on angiography, 39% had creatinine clearances (CrCl) <60 ml/min [11]. This dual organ dysfunction is now termed *the cardiorenal syndrome* (CRS).

CRS describes interactions between the cardiovascular and renal systems in which therapy to ameliorate congestive heart failure is limited by deleterious effects on renal function and hemodynamics. The classification, proposed by Ronco *et al.* [12], includes 5 subtypes:

Type 1: Acute CHF resulting in acute kidney injury (AKI)
Type 2: Chronic (progressive) cardiac dysfunction resulting in CKD

Type 3: Acute and often abrupt deterioration in renal function resulting in acute cardiac dysfunction

Type 4: Primary CKD contributing to worsening cardiac dysfunction

Type 5: Acute or chronic systemic disorders that cause both cardiac and renal dysfunction (such as sepsis, endocarditis, or diabetes mellitus)

In this review we focus on CRS type 2, which, in addition to its therapy-limiting physiology, is often associated with diuretic resistance and refractory disease [13]. In such cases, prescribing drugs inhibiting the renin-angiotensin system may risk precipitating further declines in kidney function, and patients may experience symptoms of volume overload that is refractory to diuretics. Hypervolemia is the target of much of this focus in CHF management, and ultimately, an alternate means of fluid removal must be available for these patients.

In 1949, Schneierson published the first case report documenting the successful use of peritoneal ultrafiltration to treat CHF refractory to conventional therapy [14]. This modality for optimizing volume management has several potential advantages. In the outpatient dialysis setting, peritoneal dialysis (PD) is often a preferred choice due to gradual, slow ultrafiltration. Likely for this reason, PD is associated with the preservation of residual renal function, and additionally, patients are able to perform their own treatments outside the hospital setting associated with a better quality of life. In addition there is the theoretical advantage of clearance of proinflammatory cytokines and humoral factors that may contribute to myocardial depression and progression of cardiovascular dysfunction. All of these qualities make PD an excellent modality for renal replacement therapy (RRT) and volume management.

Unfortunately, there were early difficulties surrounding technique failure and infection associated with PD catheters. Since those early attempts, PD technology has improved with advances such as closed loop fill and drain bag systems, double cuffed tunneled catheters and peritoneal tube exit site antibiotic prophylaxis. Numerous case reports and series have demonstrated success in treating hypervolemia with PD, independent of the advances in CHF pharmacotherapy. Patients having receiving this therapy have demonstrated: improving increasing left ventricular systolic function [15-19], improved diuretic-responsiveness [20,21], preservation and stability of renal function, improved functional class [15-25,27-30], decreased hospitalization [21,22,31], and improved quality of life [29]. The impact on mortality remains unclear, as virtually all case patients have had significantly limited life expectancy related to severe CHF and associated comorbid conditions.

New technologies such as peripheral ultrafiltration (UF) also offer a gentle approach to volume removal. Peripheral UF is performed in a hospital setting via peripheral venous catheter, removing essentially isotonic/iso-osmotic plasma water from whole blood at rates ranging from 10-500mL per hour, with pump speeds of 10-40mL/minute, and in some cases only requiring 33mL of extracorporeal blood volume at any given time. There is preliminary evidence of its efficacy as demonstrated in the UNLOAD Trial by Costanzo *et al.* [32]. In this study, 200 patients were randomized to either standard care (including intravenous diuretics) or peripheral UF for the management of hypervolemic heart failure requiring hospitalization. At 90 days, patients assigned to UF had a significantly decreased re-hospitalization rate compared to standard treatment (0.22 versus 0.46 admissions per patient, p=0.022), decreased days in hospital (1.4 ± 4.2 versus 3.8 ±8.5, p=0.022), and a decreased number of unscheduled physician visits (21% versus 44%, p=0.009). There were similar changes in serum creatinine in both groups, and there was no correlation between net fluid removal and increased serum creatinine.

In this review, we aim to examine the evidence for PD use in CHF. Specifically, we will review the existing literature outlining the populations studied and their outcomes both PD-related (peritonitis, technique failure) and non-PD-related (mortality, hospitalizations, quality of life).

Methodology

We conducted a literature search of Medline through PubMed (1945 – April 2011), Scopus, Summons and Cochrane databases initially using the terms "peritoneal dialysis" and "heart failure." The MeSH database resulted in 173 articles, of which 19 were considered relevant. The Summons database resulted in 7718 articles, of which 11 were selected. Subsequently, each of the terms "mortality," "hospitalization," "quality of life", and "infection," was combined in various permutations with the Medical Subject Heading terms "peritoneal dialysis" and "heart failure." All articles were then reviewed manually to identify as many case reports and series of patients in whom peritoneal dialysis was used as a modality to treat congestive heart failure. Review articles were also considered for additional information. In total, 20 case reports and series were identified and retrieved.

PATHOPHYSIOLOGY OF CHF

CHF is a complex process involving cardiac, neurohumoral, and renal mechanisms, ultimately resulting in ventricular remodeling, decreased effective cardiac output, and progressive CKD secondary to renal hypoperfusion. As ventricular function becomes less efficient, there are compensatory increases in heart rate, systemic vascular resistance, and preload. Activation of the renin-angiotensin-aldosterone system (RAAS) and release of vasopressin leads to increased sodium and water reclamation as well as a compensatory response in vascular tone. With the increases in volume, preload, and afterload, cardiac output is maintained at the expense of an increased myocardial oxygen demand and further cardiac remodeling. Eventually, these neurohumoral mechanisms lead to hypervolemia, hyponatremia, persistently impaired cardiac output, and a decline in glomerular filtration rate (GFR).

The current mainstays of therapy for systolic heart failure are aimed at counteracting the pathologic mechanisms and breaking the cycle facilitated by activation of the RAAS. Diuretics, preload and afterload reduction, and aldosterone antagonists comprise the bulk of pharmacologic intervention in the majority of heart failure patients. Despite this, cardiac function does tend to deteriorate, and as CHF becomes more severe, diuretic resistance may also ensue.

INDICATIONS FOR PD IN CHF

No clear, objective criteria for the initiation of PD (or any form of RRT) for the treatment of CHF have been established. PD has been used as a) a transient therapy to improve volume overload and possibly increase diuretic-responsiveness; b) a temporizing measure to bridge a patient to more definitive therapy, such as valve repair/replacement or cardiac transplantation; or c) as a continuous therapy for patients with refractory disease and are poor candidates for other therapies. The literature reports PD utilization in patients with severe, symptomatic volume overload refractory to therapy with intravenous diuretics and without contraindications to peritoneal ultrafiltration. Additionally, there is no clear definition of diuretic failure in terms of dose, route administered, diuretic class and quantification of urine output.

From early reports to the present, the primary indication for PD in the management of CHF has been symptomatic, hypervolemic heart failure that is refractory to standard therapy. Of note, there is significant variability in therapeutic choices utilized in the available literature, including the use of sodium and fluid restriction, angiotensin receptor inhibition and blockade, varying doses of diuretics (the majority of which are loop diuretics and aldosterone antagonists), and inotropes such as digoxin. Some contemporary studies also comment on management of anemia and cardiac resyn chronization therapy (CRT) [21, 29]. The definition of refractory disease or diuretic resistance is clinician-dependent, as has been the decision to pursue extracorporeal methods of fluid removal. There have been no head-to head randomized control trials comparing PD to intravenous diuretics or to hemodialysis (HD) for CHF management. Additionally, there have been no trials of initiation of PD for mild to moderate CHF that we are aware of.

Patients described in the current literature tend to be older (with some exception), have significant functional limitation, severely impaired cardiac function, and some degree of renal failure (many studies quoted serum creatinine concentrations and GFRs consistent with stage 3-5 CKD). Additionally, a high level of overall morbidity and severely decreased life expectancy was universal. As an example, a study by Gotloib *et al.* specifically reviewed patients that were virtually certain not to be transplant candidates [28]. Of the literature examined for this review, 116 patients out of 153 commenced PD for primary cardiac indications with associated non-ESRD CKD, and the remainder had ESRD requiring renal replacement therapy (RRT). 54 patients were given either conventional HD or UF prior to PD (either to treat acute volume overload, facilitate body wall optimization for PD catheter placement, or both) [17, 20, 21, 28, 29, and 33]. Tormey *et al.* used responsiveness to continuous veno-venous hemofiltration (CVVH) to enroll 3 of 5 patients for fluid management with PD, postulating that the absence of response to CVVH would predict poor response to other forms of ultrafiltration [22]. None of the patients reviewed were documented as having normal renal function. There was representation from both sexes. Though nephrology and cardiology practices vary between regions, experience with this modality was noted in North America, Europe, the Middle East, and Japan [17, 21, 19, and 27].

In earlier literature (1960's and 1970's), intermittent PD was utilized. Generally speaking, reports showed an improvement in functional capacity, decreased total body water, increased diuretic-responsiveness [34, 35], improvement in hyponatremia and pulmonary capillary wedge pressure [36].

Unfortunately, many of those studies were associated with a relatively high incidence of catheter infection, catheter leaking, and peritonitis.

In the 1980's, reports of continuous ambulatory PD (CAPD) emerged, and as PD components and techniques improved, complication rates began to decline. In a study by McKinnie *et al.* in 1985 and a later study by Konig *et al.* in 1987, a total of 5 patients had no PD complications, no reported admissions for CHF exacerbations, and their functional capacities all improved [24,30]. Conversely, Rubin and Ball noted no significant change in hospitalization, and indicated peritonitis and myocardial infarction as admission diagnoses in their patients [18]. Of note, they stated that CAPD was not associated with excessive rates of peritonitis, though the incidence in their study was not reported. Additionally, they described improved diuretic responsiveness in a patient such that PD was ceased. Since then, other reports have documented an improvement in diuretic response as well.

In several reported cases, patients with end stage renal disease (ESRD) on HD have been converted to peritoneal dialysis. Hébert *et al.* described 17 patients that were started on PD, 3 of who were converted from hemodialysis to PD because of intractable angina pectoris and recurrent hypotension during dialysis sessions [16]. There was no report of hypotensive episodes after PD initiation. In addition, 2 of 17 patients survived to kidney transplantation.

OUTCOMES

No randomized control trials have been performed to date looking at survival with and without dialysis in patients with refractory CHF. Furthermore, one dialysis modality has not been proven superior to another, and oftentimes modality decisions are influenced by the acuity of renal failure. The numerous patients that present acutely are most often treated with HD, thus increasing their likelihood to be maintained on that modality. Anecdotally, many patients falling into this cohort are elderly, have numerous comorbidities, functional limitation, and relative contraindications to PD. For these reasons, patients are often deemed not to be candidates for PD. In programs optimized to deliver PD efficiently to more marginal patients with bedside placed catheters available for immediate use and home care assisted automated PD, many of these patients would be eligible.

Outcomes reviewed include: improvement in NYHA functional class, mortality, and change in left ventricular ejection fraction (LVEF), improvement in quality of life (QOL), hospitalization (secondary to PD or CHF) and complications (PD-related).

PD in patients with CHF and ESRD

There are no randomized controlled trials comparing HD and PD in ESRD patients with severe CHF. There is, however, significant overlap between both diseases; the HEMO study found that the incidence of congestive heart failure in dialysis is > 30% [37]. Prior to this, there was very little data on the epidemiology of heart failure in CKD, and it was Parfrey *et al.* that noted the prevalence of LV hypertrophy varied according to GFR: 27% with GFR of 50 ml/min, 31% with GFR of 25-49 ml/min, and 45% in those with a GFR<25 ml/min, with a 74% incidence of LVH overall [38]. In their epidemiological study, Parfrey and Foley also noted a 7.6% per year incidence of *de novo* CHF in patients after starting dialysis, with an annual incidence of 3.6% per year [38, 39], and found a dismal 5-year survival rate in ESRD patients with systolic dysfunction.

In the Hébert *et al.* study of 17 patients with ESRD and CHF in whom PD was initiated, 13 were NYHA functional class 3 or 4, while the remaining 4 patients were class 2 [16]. At the end of the study (mean follow-up 24 months), 94% of patients were class 2 or better. In terms of mortality, they noticed a similar trend towards improvement using actuarial survival rates. Rates for the study patients after initiation of PD were noted to be 94%, 30%, and 64% at 12, 18, and 24 months, respectively. This was improved when compared to matched epidemiologic data of the same period for patients with either ESRD or CHF alone. 10 patients underwent a second echocardiogram and LVEF increased from a mean value of 23.2% ± 9.1% to a mean value of 30.3% ± 8.1%, representing a 30% improvement ($P < 0.01$). In 408.4 patient-months of follow-up, there were 25 admissions in 8 patients with peritonitis, and 9 exit site infections. Of note, all of these complications occurred prior to the introduction of the PD Y-connector to the study in 1987. The Y-connector subsequently resulted in a significant decrease in peritonitis rate, admission rate, and hospitalization rate ($p<0.05$). There were 2 admissions with CHF, 1 before and 1 after 1987. No objective measure of QOL was made, but improvement was inferred (as it has been in other studies) by the significant improvement in NYHA class.

In a paper by Takane *et al.*, 124 patients started PD for the purposes of renal replacement in the study period [19]. Of those, 16 were subsequently noted to have impaired left ventricular systolic function on echocardiogram

(31% ± 3%). 12 of the patients had NYHA class 3 heart failure, and the remainder were NYHA class 2. Over the course of 12 months of CAPD, all patients experienced an improvement in their NYHA class ($p<0.01$). There were no deaths at 1 year and no patients were converted to HD. In terms of LVEF, there was a statistically significant improvement to 44% ± 6% ($p<0.05$). There was no disclosure of complications or hospitalizations.

In Kagan's review of 3 patients, a 17-year old female patient was noted to have ESRD secondary to biopsy-proven IgA nephropathy, with an associated LVEF of 55% [33]. She had been on HD for 32 months, and despite an adequate Kt/V, her cardiac function declined to 25%. She eventually required mechanical ventilation for severe pulmonary edema, and PD was initiated at that time. Over the course of 18 months of PD with 1.5% dextrose (2L x 4 exchanges daily), her functional status improved, and she qualified for kidney transplant. Subsequent measurements of LVEF were 60%.

In summary, the current data, though limited, is suggestive that PD is an appropriate mode of renal replacement therapy in the ESRD population with heart failure. The volume management and simultaneous treatment of uremia confers 2 essential therapies, with limited risk for complications and avoidance of rapid changes in metabolic parameters.

PD in patients with CHF without ESRD

There have been several small studies of patients with CHF who were administered PD for the primary goal of volume management. In several cases, IPD has been used as a rescue therapy. When not in the context of ESRD, diuretic resistance and refractory heart failure is an indication for ultrafiltration. By removing excess volume, improvement of oxygenation, respiratory mechanics, and cardiac output should follow. As with CVVH, PD has the advantage over HD of being slower and continuous, assuaging rapid fluid shifts and avoiding wide changes in preload or afterload. Additionally, continuous convection results in satisfactory correction of hyponatremia and adequate removal of fluid. Lastly, PD offers significant latitude in tailoring therapy to each individual. Limitations include difficulty in catheter placement in the acute setting (immaturity of the catheter, and significant body wall edema), and pericatheter leaks. Recent data suggests pericatheter leaks can be avoided by instilling low volumes of dialysate. [25].

There is more experience with PD in the chronic management of refractory heart failure, the vast sum of which is derived from case reports and series. Overall, most studies since 1985 created various regimens of CAPD for their patients, with dwell times and tonicity titrated for fluid removal between 0.5-2L per day.

Gotloib and colleagues in 2005 reported 20 patients with NYHA class 4 heart failure who were considered for various reasons not to be candidates for cardiac transplantation, and thus were started on PD [28]. Initially, they were treated with CVVH to improve volume status and body wall characteristics prior to PD catheter placement, and then started on 3 APD sessions/week x 8hrs each, with 15–20L of dialysis fluid/session using 10.35±3.05L of 1.5% lactated glucose and 8.95 ±2.95L of 4.25% glucose. Subsequently, they were maintained on APD 3/week x 8 hours. Mean ultrafiltration rate was 2102±505 mL/session. The investigators found that total days in hospital after PD was initiated fell from 157 to 13 in the post-intervention period ($p<0.001$). Additionally, he found that all patients were relieved of their class 4 symptomatology (all 20 improving to NYHA class 1). Of particular note is the study's mortality rate; the study patients received a mean Charlson's comorbidity index of 7.8±1.8, with a range of 6-13. A score > 5 foretells a poor prognosis, and predicts a mortality rate of 85% within 1 year. Of the 20 patients included in the study, the mortality rate was only 10% at 1 year, and 20% at 396 patient-months. This suggests PD may offer a significant benefit not only in terms of functional class, but also in terms of mortality. There are, however, several limitations. Adjunctive therapies that may or may not have influenced survival (such as anti-arrhythmics or CRT) were not disclosed. There were no complications disclosed with respect to PD technique or infection, though the authors' substantially lower hospitalization rate suggests few problems. Additionally, the causes of death in this study were not reviewed.

A promising study was published in 2010 by Cnossen *et al.*, involving 24 patients who were progressing towards ESRD (mean GFR 14.8mL ± 12.1mL) and had concomitant systolic dysfunction (mean EF 33% ± 16%) [31]. All patients received commercially available glucose or icodextran dialysate; 6 patients were started on a single dwell per day, and the remainder were initiated on 4 dwells of 2L per 24 hours. At the end of one year, there was a significant decrease in hospitalization for cardiovascular causes (3.7 ± 3.8 predialysis vs. 1.4 ± 2.1 days/patient/month postdialysis, $p = 0.041$). Median survival was 1 year. Interestingly, when comparing the cohort of patients that survived beyond 1 year to those that died prior to the median survival time, Cnossen found that there was a significant difference in all-cause hospitalizations (13.7 ± 26.5 predialysis vs. 3.5 ± 8.8 days/patient/month postdialysis, $p = 0.001$). Survivors were also younger and fewer were diabetic, but there was no significant difference in LVEF. This data is highly suggestive that PD may confer a mortality benefit in a significant cohort of individuals with heart failure, in addition to its demonstrated symptom improvement. It is also one of the largest reports of icodextrin-based therapy in this population, which, by its extended length of action and gentle fluid removal may be the most physiologically ideal therapeutic choice in CHF patients. Further study of icodextrin in this population may show potential.

OUTCOMES

NYHA Functional Class/ Quality of Life (QOL)

Most case reports and series document an improvement in NYHA functional class in the majority of their patients with PD in this patient population. Additionally, several authors report a subjective improvement in quality of life. Many have inferred an improvement in QOL based on decreased hospitalization rates, improved NYHA class, a low risk of complications related to therapy, and decreased pharmacologic requirements. In 2010, Sanchez *et al.* evaluated health related quality of life using the generic EQ-5D tool [29]. A health utility score was calculated, as compared to data from individuals receiving conservative therapy, defined as drug therapy, cardiac resynchronization as indicated, hospitalization and mortality rates in patients with refractory congestive HF not treated with PD. They found a higher perceived state of health in those treated with PD ($p < 0.01$).

Improvements and measurement dilemmas in left ventricular function

Changes to LVEF have been heterogeneous, with Bertoli *et al.* and Prochnicka and her colleagues showing a substantial increases in EF, from 25% to 50% and 40% to 55%, respectively (each in 1 patient) [15,17]. In Hébert's review of 17 patients, 10 of whom had a repeat echocardiogram after PD was initiated; there was an increase in LVEF from a mean value of 23.2% ± 9.1% to a mean value of 30.3% ± 8.1% ($P < 0.01$). Of note, only 1 patient in his study reached an EF greater than 30%. In 2006, Takane *et al.* also found an improved LVEF, from 31% ± 3% to 44% ± 6% ($p<0.01$) [19]. Despite these studies' trends towards improved systolic function, there is conflicting data.

In 1998, Ryckelynck *et al.* noted that of the 7 patients that had repeat systolic function measurement, only 3 improved, while 2 remained stable and

2 declined [23]. In 2009, Basile *et al.* found that only 1 of 4 patients had an improved EF, while 2 remained stable, and the last actually deteriorated despite an improvement in symptoms [20]. They specifically noted no association between improvement in EF and symptomatology. Both studies noted a universal improvement in NYHA class. The Sanchez *et al.* 2010 study had similar results; though there was a significant improvement in functional class in all ($p<0.001$) and associated decrease in hospitalization, there was no associated improvement in LVEF [29].

It then stands that the reasons for heterogeneity in LVEF response are multifactorial. While many patients' hearts have undergone fixed ventricular remodeling, there are a subset of patients whose hearts are able to recover systolic function. One possible explanation is the effects of fluid overload via the Frank-Starling mechanism impair the dynamic function of the heart, and fluid removal unmasks residual systolic function. It must be noted that improvement in LVEF in these studies is not associated with improved survival or improved functional capacity, and it may stand to reason that increased systolic function may be beneficial, or may also be detrimental by way of increasing myocardial oxygen demand on an already taxed heart.

By the same token, the heterogeneity in cutoffs for what entails "left ventricular dysfunction" poses a dilemma. Timing of ventricular assessment and mode of LVEF measurement must be considerations [40].

Current recommendations for the classification of EF stratify dysfunction as mild (LVEF – 41-49%), moderate (LVEF – 35–40%) and severe (LVEF < 35%) [41]. Definitions of what is deemed *significant* LVEF impairment are inconsistent (in the studies reviewed in this review as well as in others), thus resulting in variable study populations. This characteristic further thwarts attempts for combined analyses of different study populations. The large cohort study of left ventricular dysfunction in ESRD by Parfrey *et al.* [38] used a cutoff ejection fraction of 25% versus a comparable study by Mallamaci *et al.* that used 40% [42]. Interestingly, despite the lower cutoff, the Parfrey group reported a higher prevalence of systolic dysfunction as compared to the Mallamaci group (16% versus 13%). This result may be explained in part by the timing of the echocardiogram [40].

In Mallamaci's study population, echocardiography took place midweek. In Parfrey's patient population, timing of echocardiography was not specified; it may have in fact been pre-dialysis, thus resulting in an underestimation of true LV function [40]. With this in mind, it is essential to acknowledge the potential for error inherent with echocardiography. As described above, the most widely used means of measurement of left ventricular function is M mode, two-dimensional echocardiography. It is one of the most commonly utilized modality of diagnosing LV dysfunction. While its benefits include wide availability, relatively low cost and good inter-observer reliability [43], errors may occur because many of the measurements are indirect; they are extrapolated based on geometric assumptions that hold true for most, but not all patients.

As an example, the echocardiographic calculated left ventricular mass (LVM) relies heavily on measurement of left ventricular internal dimension (LVID) that, in turn, is susceptible to changes with plasma volume [43]. Clearly, volume status at the time of echocardiography is paramount to obtaining an accurate measure. Failure to obtain a true dry weight prior to echocardiogram – or echocardiography prior to HD – leads to underestimations of LV function. This was demonstrated in two small series in which the average reductions in LVMI and end diastolic diameter from pre- to postdialysis were 26.2–36.1 g/m2 and 4–8.4 mm, respectively [44,45].

Newer techniques of visualization of cardiac structures are emerging that may minimize this information bias. Cardiac magnetic resonance imaging (cMRI) directly measures cardiac mass, thereby circumventing the geometric assumptions and calculations used in echocardiography. In a head to head comparison of cMRI versus echocardiography in the HD population, echocardiography overestimated LVM compared to cMRI, which detected lower LV mass (193.2 versus 122.3 g/m2 for men, 133.5 versus 89.6 g/m2 for women) and had better intra-observer variability (4.3% versus 9.6%) [46]. Of note, the same study found that as left ventricular dilatation increased, the overestimation of LVM by echocardiography also increased in a linear fashion. Cardiac MRI is limited by cost, availability, claustrophobia, contraindications such as pacemakers, as well as concerns with gadolinium use (in infused studies) and the associated potential for nephrogenic systemic fibrosis. Despite this, its accuracy, increasing utility, and improved availability suggest it as a promising technology. Alternately, real-time 3D echocardiography (RT3DE) and cardiac CT (CCT) are also potential modalities for cardiac structural assessment.

Mortality

Mortality, as has previously been discussed, is difficult to study in this population. Decreased mortality noted by Gotloib's group raises hope that PD may have a modest effect on survival [28]. In the subsequent study by Sanchez and colleagues, all 17 patients had symptomatic heart failure and GFRs that ranged between 15mL/min and 68mL/min (mean – 35mL/min) [29]. Patients were followed for 15 ± 9 months and the authors were able to note an increase in life expectancy (82% after 12 months of treatment, and 70% and 56% after 18 and 24 months respectively). Of interest, these patients were aggressively treated with other modalities as well. They received diuretics, angiotensin receptor and beta-adrenergic antagonists, digoxin (if in atrial fibrillation), phosphodiesterase therapy if pulmonary hypertension existed, and cardiac resynchronization therapy (CRT) if deemed appropriate.

Hospitalization for heart failure

Within most studies, there was a statistically significant decrease in hospitalization. Rubin and Ball reported no significant change in hospitalization, and indicated peritonitis and myocardial infarction as main admission diagnoses in their population [18]. Of note, they stated that CAPD was not associated with excessive peritonitis (as compared to standard rates of the era). There were no admissions with acute exacerbations of CHF in the follow-up period. Since this report, numerous studies have had similar findings. Tormey *et al.* found hospitalization decreased by 85% in their series of 3 patients [22]. Gotloib *et al.* noted a decrease from 157 days in hospital to 13 days before and after PD was initiated [28], and Sanchez' group noted a decrease from 62 ± 16 days/patient/year to 11 ± 5 days/patient/year (p=0.003) before and after PD treatment, respectively [29]. Only Ryckelynck reported a rate of complications of which CHF comprised 36% of the reasons for admission [23]. Despite this, the overall lower hospitalization rate has been reproducible and encouraging.

PD-related complications

PD-related complications have declined in all populations, having been ameliorated by new catheter connectology, automation, improved peritonitis infection prophylaxis and reduced touch contamination. Generally speaking, the rates of PD-related complications are low, and do not appear to pose excess risk to patients. Of the reports we reviewed, multiple investigators did not note any specific PD-associated complications [15, 17, 20, 22, 27, and 28].

In 1995, Hébert's group noted that 8 of their 17 patients had 25 episodes of peritonitis cumulatively, requiring 14 hospital admissions [16]. In addition, there were 9 exit site infections (ESI). Interestingly, all episodes of peritonitis and ESI that required admission to hospital occurred prior to the introduction of the Y-connector into patients' PD apparatus ($p<0.05$). In 1998, Ryckelyck published a high rate of complications as well [23]; 16% of complications were related to PD: skin infection (n=1), peritonitis (n=2), transient lack of drainage (n=3), and catheter displacement requiring replacement (n=2).

In the most recent literature, Cnossen *et al.* found few PD technique complications in their 24 patients [31], including: pericatheter leakage (n = 1), recurrent peritonitis (n = 2), and umbilical hernia (n = 1). Nakayama *et al.* had 1 death secondary to catheter-related peritonitis [21]. Sanchez' group found that peritonitis was present but rare in their population as there were only 0.02 episodes /patient/year at risk, which is lower than their local PD registry rate of 0.56 episodes/patient/year at risk ($p=0.008$) [29].

There was only 1 admission with hypotension secondary to excessive ultrafiltration [17]. This was related to a miscalculation in dialysate concentration by the patient and did not result in long term sequelae.

Other findings

2 studies in particular looked at other metrics within their patient populations [15, 27]. Elhalel-Drantizki *et al.* found that the total number of drugs their patients require decreased from 8.1±0.7 to 5.1±0.4 in their study focusing on improving quality of life (based on improved functional class, decreased pharmacotherapy, and reduced hospitalization). Bertoli's group found increased lean body mass in their 2 patients, which suggested amelioration of cachexia and an overall improved state of health.

LIMITATIONS

There are several limitations to this data. First of all, the small numbers of patients make outcome analysis problematic. Studies of limited quantities of patients who are not responsive to the mainstays of therapy – many of whom have already reached the limit of their life expectancy – are difficult to interpret in terms of disease modification. Measurements of survival in this population are difficult due to the even higher degree of mortality inherent with concomitant heart failure and CKD. As these patients are severely limited by both CHF and CKD, this hinders not only their survival, but also their prognosis during concomitant unrelated illnesses. In many reports, therapies directed towards CHF were either not fully outlined, or incomplete (as compared to current standards that include interruption of the RAAS pathway as well as antihypertensive and statin therapy). Additionally, as therapies for many etiologies of CHF have evolved, so too have therapeutics for coronary artery disease and arrhythmias, two of the major causes of death in end-stage CHF. Lastly, it is often difficult to distinguish the myocardial depression effect of primary heart failure from that of progressive uremia and its metabolic and proinflammatory consequences, and this may confound outcomes.

The goals of management in this cohort are also important. Typically these patients are quite frail and nearing the end of life. They are often not candidates for more definitive therapy such as heart transplant, and the natural history of their disease is thus relatively fixed. Once appropriate pharmacotherapy is employed, PD may be a useful adjunctive strategy to improve quality of life and minimize hospitalization.

In summary, the currently available data must be interpreted with caution and careful speculation, and thus as it stands, PD is typically offered to those patients with heart failure and associated CKD that does not respond to evidence-based therapies.

Conclusion

The current data for the application of PD to the CHF population is limited to those with end stage cardiac disease or concomitant ESRD. Keeping this in mind, one can draw several conclusions.

The available data suggest that PD has a clear, reproducible effect on exercise tolerance and functional capacity, even in this frail population. The vast majority of patients have had documented improvements in NYHA class. As a corollary, hospitalizations have been noted to decrease in most studies. This observation was independent of any changes in LVEF, which suggests that improvement of volume overload was a main determinant of improved functional capacity. The changes to left ventricular systolic function are heterogeneous – an understandable finding, considering that significant irreversible cardiac remodeling has taken place, and that the determinants of systolic function are multivariate, depending on mechanical, nervous, renal and hormonal factors.

Changes in quality of life (QOL) have not been extensively studied. There are few objective QOL measurements in this population, though reports of individuals' experiences are described. As the population in question has a limited life expectancy, a logical measure of therapeutic efficacy would include functional capacity and QOL.

Table 1. Summary of studies reporting symptom improvement and mortality

Authors	Population (n)	Follow-up Period (average months)	Symptom Improvement (n)	Death	Comments
McKinnie *et al.* 1985 [30]	1	24months	1	Death at 24 months of MI	
Rubin and Ball 1986 [18]	8	33-1634 days	8	Median survival 225 days	No significant decrease in hospitalization
Konig *et al.* 1991 [25]	13	1.5 to 67	13	-	1 pt. underwent heart transplant
Hébert *et al.* 1995 [16]	17	24 ±17	17	5	2 patients transplanted
Tormey *et al.* 1996 [22]	3	18 ± 10	3	-	Hospitalization decreased
Elhalel-Dranitzki *et al.* 1998 [27]	9	> 24 months	9	5 (non-PD deaths)	Decreased pharmacotherapy 3 non-PD related sepsis 1 MI 1 sudden death
Ryckelynck *et al.* 1998 [23]	15	12.7	15	4	6 patients withdrew from the study 2 received kidney transplants
Bertoli *et al.* 2005 [15]	2	12	2	0	Increased lean body mass
Gotloib *et al.* 2005 [28]	20	7 – 35	20	10% at 1 yr. 20% at 396 patient-months	Predicted mortality was 85% pre-study based on Charlson co-morbidity score

Table 1. (Continued).

Authors	Population (n)	Follow-up Period (average months)	Symptom Improvement (n)	Death	Comments
Kagan *et al.* 2005 [33]	3	Variable	3	1 death at 14 months	Death secondary to cardiovascular collapse
Basile *et al.* 2006 [20]	4	24.3 (11-43)	4	3 (at 11, 13, 43 months)	No PD-related deaths
Takane *et al.* 2006 [19]	16	12	16	0	No deaths at 1 year
Prochnicka *et al.* 2009 [17]	1	7	1	0	1 episode of hypovolemia secondary to PD
Cnossen *et al.* 2010 [31]	24	> 1 year (August 1997 – January 2009)		4pts withdrew from PD and died 8 due to vascular disease 9 others	CV Hospitalization decreased 3.7 ± 3.8 predialysis vs. 1.4 ± 2.1 days/patient/month postdialysis, $p = 0.041$
Nakayama *et al.* 2010 [21]	12	26.5 months	12	3 non-cardiac, 1 catheter peritonitis	Diuretics withdrawn or reduced in all patients No hospitalizations during follow-up
Sanchez *et al.* 2010 [29]	17	From 2004-2008 Up to 24 months	17	1 (oropharyngeal cancer)	QOL improved perception of health (EQ-5D scale) Increased life expectancy 82% after 12 months of treatment; 70% and 56% after 18 and 24 months respectively

Table 2. Summary of studies reporting changes in the functional status as measured by the New York Heart Association (NYHA) class before and after initiation of PD

Authors	Population	NYHA Class before PD initiation	NYHA Class after PD initiation
McKinnie *et al.* 1985 [30]	1	NYHA 4 – 1 pt.	NYHA 2 – 1 pt.
Rubin and Ball 1986 [18]	8	NYHA 4 – 8 pts.	NYHA 4 – 5 pts. NYHA 3 – 3 pts.
König *et al.* 1987 [24]	4	NYHA 4 – 4 pts.	NYHA 2 – 4 pts.
König *et al.* 1991 [25]	13	NYHA 4 – 13 pts.	NYHA 2 – 13 pts.
Hébert *et al.* 1995 [16]	17	NYHA 3 or 4 –13 pts. NYHA 2 – 4 pts.	*NYHA 1 – 1 pt. NYHA 2 - 15pts NYHA 3 – 1 pt.
Tormey *et al.* 1996 [22]	3	NYHA 4 – 3 pts.	NYHA 2 – 3 pts.
Elhalel-Dranitzki *et al.* 1998 [27]	9	NYHA 4 – 9 pts.	NYHA 2.3 ± 2
Ryckelynck *et al.* 1998 [23]	15	NYHA 4 – 11 pts. NYHA 3 – 4 pts.	NYHA 3 – 4 pts. NYHA 2 – 11 pts.
Bertoli *et al.* 2005 [15]	2	NYHA 3 – 1 pt. NYHA 4 – 1 pt.	NYHA 2 – 1 pt. not noted
Gotloib *et al.* 2005 [28]	20	NYHA 4 – 20 pts.	NYHA 1 – 20 pts.
Basile *et al.* 2006 [20]	4	NYHA 4 – 4 pts.	NYHA 2.5 ±2.6 (all improved by 1 or 2 classes)
Takane *et al.* 2006 [19]	16	NYHA 3 – 12 pts. NYHA 2 – 4 pts.	NYHA 2 – 11 pts. NYHA 1 – 5 pts.
Prochnicka *et al.* 2009 [17]	1	NYHA 4 – 1 pt.	NYHA 1/2 – 1 pt.
Nakayama *et al.* 2010 [21]	12	NYHA 3 – 9 pts. NYHA 4 – 3 pts.	NYHA 1 – 9 pts. NYHA 2 – 3 pts.
Sanchez *et al.* 2010 [29]	17	NYHA 4 – 10 pts. NYHA 3 – 7 pts.	NYHA 3 – 1 pt. NYHA 2 – 13 pts. NYHA 1 – 3 pts. (11 pts. improved 2 classes, 6 improved 1 class)

*at 6 months

Table 3. Summary table of studies describing PD regiment, modality, ultrafiltration and complications

Authors	Population	PD regimen	Ultrafiltration rate	Complications
McKinnie *et al.* 1985 [30]	1	CAPD 4.25% dextrose. 2-3 exchanges/day.	500mL – 1500mL per day	No PD complications
Rubin and Ball 1986 [18]	8	Variable concentrations of dextrose	-	
König *et al.* 1987 [24]	4	CAPD 4.25% dextrose	-	No PD complications
König *et al.* 1991 [25]	13	CAPD 1.5% or 4.25% hydrous dextrose; dialysate concentration was chosen by the investigator or patient individually to attain control of body water. Titrated to a maximum of 2L, while the number of fluid exchanges was reduced from 6 to 3 per day.	Not noted	
Hébert *et al.* 1995 [16]	17	4 daily 1.5L - 2.5L exchanges with 1.5%, 2.58%, or 4.25% dextrose dialysate (individually adjusted)	Not noted	8 patients accounted for 25 episodes of peritonitis and 9 exit site infections
Tormey *et al.* 1996 [22]	3	1.5 or 2L of glucose 1.36% or 3.86% dialysate, (individually adjusted) Dwell time of 2-4h	Not noted	None noted
Elhalel-Dranitzki *et al.* 1998 [27]	9	CAPD	–	No PD complications
Ryckelynck *et al.* 1998 [23]	15	Various regimens Dianeal dextrose 3.86% or 1.36% One hypertonic bag q24hrs for 7 pts. One hypertonic bag q48hrs for 4 pts. Three isotonic bags per q24hrs for 1 pt. Three isotonic bags and 1 hypertonic bag per q24hrs for 2 pts.	Not noted	Hospitalizations Decreased by 67% 36% and 16% of hospitalizations were CHF and PD complications, respectively

Authors	Population	PD regimen	Ultrafiltration rate	Complications
Bertoli *et al.* 2005 [15]	2	Nocturnal exchange with icodextrin dialysate	Patient 1 – 500 cc/day Patient 2 – 1000cc/day	None related to PD or CHF
Gotloib *et al.* 2005 [28]	20	Three APD Sessions per week (8 hours each), 15–20L of dialysate per session (10.35 ± 3.05L of 1.5% lactated glucose and 8.95 ± 2.95L of 4.25% glucose)	Average – 2102mL ± 505 mL per session	No complications disclosed
Basile *et al.* 2006 [20]	4	Icodextrin dialysate 1 nocturnal exchange with icodextrin in 3 patients 2 exchanges in 1 patient (icodextrin + 1.36% isotonic dextrose solution)	Range 409mL – 2379mL per day	No episodes of peritonitis
Takane *et al.* 2006 [19]	16	Four daily 2L exchanges using 1.5% or 2.5% dextrose	Not noted	-
Prochnicka *et al.* 2009 [17]	1	2 daytime exchanges with 1.36% glucose dialysate, 1 overnight exchange with icodextrin	Average – 1970 ± 500 mL	
Cnossen *et al.* 2010 [31]	24	Glucose and icodextrin dialysate. 6 patients started initially with 1 dwell per day (incremental CAPD). Other patients started with 4 dwells of 2L per 24hours.	–	PD technique - 17% Pericatheter leakage (n = 1) Recurrent peritonitis (n = 2) Umbilical hernia (n = 1)
Nakayama *et al.* 2010 [21]	12	Sequential HF prior to starting PD, then 3 times per week x 8hours, titrated as indicated	-	1 catheter related peritonitis
Sanchez *et al.* 2010 [29]	17	Variable regimens with icodextrin	Average – 670mL ± 225mL per session	6 of 17 initially needed venous ultrafiltration

Complications associated with PD appear to be minimal, with peritonitis as well as catheter-tip/cutaneous infections comprising the majority of these few complications. There was only 1 case of significant symptomatic hypovolemia related to PD [17], and in this case it was a calculation error made by the patient in terms of dialysate concentration. Overall, the data suggests that PD is at least as safe in the CHF population as in those with ESRD as a primary indication.

Conclusions as they apply to mortality are difficult because 1) of the aforementioned age and severity of disease of the currently studied patients, 2) the relatively small numbers of patients in which PD is considered a therapeutic option for CHF, and 3) the associated high risk of death from comorbid states. As noted by Cnossen et al, age appears to be a prognostic factor for survival past 1 year [31]. Thus, it may prove worthwhile to review the outcomes of younger patients offered this modality. As noted in the same paper, diabetes mellitus appears to be a negative prognosticator. Limiting patients by comorbidities may also uncover a beneficial effect on mortality in a subset. Studies demonstrating these hypotheses have yet to be done.

PD is a well-recognized modality of volume management that has demonstrated clear effects on patients' level of function. As a slow-acting method of fluid removal, it approximates physiologic diuresis, and avoids some of the pitfalls of hemodialysis and aggressive diuretic strategies. Its utility in the outpatient setting creates less disruption in patients' day-to-day lives, and decreases the number of days in hospital. The optimal timing of initiation of PD has yet to be determined, although it stands to reason that mortality-altering therapy should be initiated and optimized first.

REFERENCES

[1] Bristow MR, Gilbert EM, Abraham WT, Adams KF, Fowler MB, Hershberger RE, Kubo SH, Narahara KA, Ingersoll H, Krueger, Young S, Shusterman N. Carvedilol produces dose-related improvements in left ventricular function and survival in subjects with chronic heart failure. MOCHA Investigators. Circulation 1996; 94:2807-16.

[2] Kjekshus J, Swedberg K, Snapinn S. Effects of enalapril on long-term mortality in severe congestive heart failure. CONSENSUS Trial Group. Am J Cardiol 1992; 69:103-7?

[3] The SOLVD Investigators. Effect of enalapril on survival in patients with reduced left ventricular ejection fractions and congestive heart failure. N Engl J Med 1991; 325: 293-302.

[4] Pitt B, Zannad F, Remme WJ, Cody R, Castaigne A, Perez A, Palensky J, Wittes J. The effect of spironolactone on morbidity and mortality in patients with severe heart failure. Randomized Aldactone Evaluation Study Investigators. N Engl J Med 1999; 341:709-17.

[5] Brandimarte F, Fedele F, De Luca L, Fonarow GC, Gheorghiade M. Hyponatremia in acute heart failure syndromes: a potential therapeutic target. Curr Heart Fail Rep. 2007 Dec; 4(4):207-13.

[6] Waikar SS, Curhan GC, Brunelli SM. Mortality associated with low serum sodium concentration in maintenance hemodialysis. Am J Med. 2011 Jan; 124(1):77-84.

[7] Whelan B, Bennett K, O'Riordan D, Silke B. Serum sodium as a risk factor for in-hospital mortality in acute unselected general medical patients. Q J Med 2009; 102:175–182.

[8] Foley RN, Parfrey PS, Harnett JD, Kent GM, Martin CJ, Murray DC, Barre PE. Clinical and echocardiographic disease in patients starting end-stage renal disease therapy. Kidney Int 1995; 47: 1861–1892.

[9] Harnett JD, Foley RN, Kent GM, Barre PE, Murray D, Parfrey PS. Congestive heart failure in dialysis patients: prevalence, incidence, prognosis and risk factors. Kidney Int 1995; 47: 884–890.

[10] Adams KF Jr, Fonarow GC, Emerman CL, LeJemtel TH, Costanzo MR, Abraham, Berkowitz RL, Galvao M, Horton DP; ADHERE Scientific Advisory Committee and Investigators. Characteristics and outcomes of patients hospitalized for heart failure in the United States: rationale, design, and preliminary observations from the first 100 000 cases in the Acute Decompensated Heart Failure National Registry (ADHERE). Am Heart J 2005; 149: 209–216.

[11] Ezekowitz J, McAlister FA, Humphries KH, Norris CM, Tonelli M, Ghali WA, Knudtson ML; APPROACH Investigators. The association among renal insufficiency, pharmacotherapy, and outcomes in 6427 patients with heart failure and coronary artery disease. J Am Coll Cardiol 2004; 44: 1587-1592.

[12] Ronco C, Haapio M, House , Anavekar N, Bellomo R. Cardiorenal syndrome. J Am Coll Cardiol. 2008; 52: 1527-1539.

[13] Ronco C, Ricci Z, Bellomo R, Bedogni F. Extracorporeal ultrafiltration for the treatment of overhydration and congestive heart failure. Cardiology 2001; 96: 155–168

[14] Shneierson SJ. Continuous peritoneal irrigation in the treatment of intractable edema of cardiac origin. Am J Med Sci. 1949; 218: 76-79.
[15] Bertoli SV, Ciurlino D, Maccario M, Martino S, Bigatti G, Traversi L, Procaccio M, Buzzi L. Home peritoneal ultrafiltration in patients with severe congestive heart failure without end-stage renal disease. Adv Perit Dial. 2005;21:123-7.
[16] Hébert MJ, Falardeau M, Pichette V, Houde M, Nolin L, Cardinal J, Ouimet D. Continuous ambulatory peritoneal dialysis Am J Kidney Dis. 1995 May; 25(5):761-8.
[17] Próchnicka A, Olszowska A, Baczyński D, Zelichowski G, Lubas A, Wiśniewska M, Dziekiewicz M, Wańkowicz Z. Peritoneal dialysis Pol Arch Med Wewn. 2009 Dec;119(12):834-7.
[18] Rubin J, Ball R. Continuous ambulatory peritoneal dialysis as treatment of severe congestive heart failure in the face of chronic renal failure. Report of eight cases. Arch Intern Med. 1986 Aug;146(8):1533-5.
[19] Takane H, Nakamoto H, Arima H, Shoda J, Moriwaki K, Ikeda N, Kobayashi K, Kanno Y, Sugahara S, Okada H, Suzuki H. Continuous ambulatory peritoneal dialysis is effective for patients with severe congestive heart failure. Adv Perit Dial. 2006;22:141-6.
[20] Basile C, Chimienti D, Bruno A, Cocola S, Libutti P, Teutonico A, Cazzato F. Efficacy of peritoneal dialysis with icodextrin in the long-term treatment of refractory congestive heart failure. Perit Dial Int. 2009 Jan-Feb;29(1):116-8.
[21] Nakayama M, Nakano H, Nakayama M. Novel therapeutic option for refractory heart failure in elderly patients with chronic kidney disease by incremental peritoneal dialysis. J Cardiol. 2010 Jan;55(1):49-54. Epub 2009 Sep 26.
[22] Tormey V, Conlon PJ, Farrell J, Horgan J, Walshe JJ. Long-term successful management of refractory congestive cardiac failure by intermittent ambulatory peritoneal ultrafiltration. QJM 1996; 89:681-3.
[23] Ryckelynck JP, Lobbedez T, Valette B, Le Goff C, Mazouz O, Levaltier B, Potier JC, Hurault de Ligny B. Peritoneal ultrafiltration and treatment-resistant heart failure. Nephrol Dial Transplant. 1998;13 Suppl 4:56-9
[24] König PS, Geissler D, Lechleitner P, Spielberger M, Dittrich P. Improved management of congestive heart failure. Use of continuous ambulatory peritoneal dialysis. Arch Intern Med. 1987 Jun;147(6):1031-4.

[25] König PS, Lhotta K, Kronenberg F, Joannidis M, Herold M. CAPD: a successful treatment in patients suffering from therapy-resistant congestive heart failure. Adv Perit Dial. 1991;7:97-101.

[26] Takane H, Nakamoto H, Arima H, Shoda J, Moriwaki K, Ikeda N, Kobayashi K, Kanno Y, Sugahara S, Okada H, Suzuki H. Continuous ambulatory peritoneal dialysis is effective for patients with severe congestive heart failure. Adv Perit Dial. 2006;22:141-6.

[27] Elhalel-Dranitzki M, Rubinger D, Moscovici A, Haviv YS, Friedlaender MM, Silver J, Popovtzer MM. CAPD to improve quality of life in patients with refractory heart failure. Nephrol Dial Transplant. 1998 Dec;13 (12):3041-2.

[28] Gotloib L, Fudin R, Yakubovich M, Vienken J. Peritoneal dialysis in refractory end-stage congestive heart failure: a challenge facing a no-win situation. Nephrol Dial Transplant. 2005 Jul;20 Suppl 7:vii32-6.

[29] Sánchez JE, Ortega T, Rodríguez C, Díaz-Molina B, Martín M, Garcia-Cueto C, Vidau P, Gago E, Ortega F. Efficacy of peritoneal ultrafiltration in the treatment of refractory congestive heart failure. Nephrol Dial Transplant (2010) 25: 605–610

[30] McKinnie JJ, Bourgeois RJ, Husserl FE. Long-term therapy for heart failure with continuous ambulatory peritoneal dialysis. Arch Intern Med 1985; 145: 1128–9.

[31] Cnossen TT, Kooman JP, Konings CJ, Uszko-Lencer NH, Leunissen KM, Van der Sande FM. Peritoneal dialysis in patients with primary cardiac failure complicated by renal failure. Blood Purif. 2010;30(2):146-52. Epub 2010 Sep 15.

[32] Costanzo MR, Guglin ME, Saltzberg MT, Jessup ML, Bart BA, Teerlink JR, Jaski BE, Fang JC, Feller ED, Haas GJ, Anderson AS, Schollmeyer MP, Sobotka PA, UNLOAD Trial Investigators. Ultrafiltration versus intravenous diuretics for patients hospitalized for acute decompensated heart failure. J Am Coll Cardiol 2007;49:675-83.

[33] Kagan A, Rapoport J. The role of peritoneal dialysis in the treatment of refractory heart failure. Nephrol Dial Transplant 2005;20:28-31.

[34] Cairns KB, Porter GA, Kloster FE, Bristow JD, Griswold HE. Clinical and hemodynamic results of peritoneal dialysis for severe cardiac failure. Am Heart J 1968;76:227-234.

[35] Mailloux LU, Swartz CD, Onesti G, Heider C, Ramirez O, Brest AN. Peritoneal dialysis for refractory congestive heart failure. JAMA 1967;199:873–878.

[36] Malach M. Peritoneal dialysis for intractable heart failure in acute myocardial infarction. Am J Cardiol 1972;29:61–63.

[37] Cheung AK, Sarnak MJ, Yan G, Berkoben M, Heyka R, Kaufman A, Lewis J, Rocco M, Toto R, Windus D, Ornt D, Levey AS; HEMO Study Group. Cardiac diseases in maintenance hemodialysis patients: results of the HEMO Study. Kidney Int 2004; 65: 2380-2389.

[38] Parfrey PS, Foley RN, Harnett JD, Kent GM, Murray DC, Barre PE. Outcome and risk factors for left ventricular disorders in chronic uraemia. Nephrol Dial Transplant 1996; 11: 1277-1285.

[39] Parfrey PS, Foley RN. The clinical epidemiology of cardiac disease in chronic renal failure. J Am Soc Nephrol 1999; 10: 1606-1615.

[40] Sood MM, Pauly RP, Rigatto C, Komenda P. Left ventricular dysfunction in the haemodialysis population. NDT Plus (2008) 4: 199-205

[41] Mahadevan G, Davis RC, Frenneaux MP, Hobbs FD, Lip GY, Sanderson JE, Davies MK. Left ventricular ejection fraction: Are the revised cut-off points for defining systolic dysfunction sufficiently evidence based? Heart 2008; 94: 426-428.

[42] Mallamaci F, Zoccali C, Tripepi G, Benedetto FA, Parlongo S, Cataliotti A, Cutrupi S, Giacone G, Bellanuova I, Stancanelli B, Malatino LS; CREED Investigators. The Cardiovascular Risk Extended Evaluation. Diagnostic potential of cardiac natriuretic peptides in dialysis patients. Kidney Int 2001; 59: 1559-1566.

[43] Kilickap M, Turhan S, Sayin T, Nergizoglu G, Kutlay S, Duman N, Rahimov U, Kumbasar D, Akgun G, Erol C. Intravascular volume dependency of left ventricular mass calculation by two-dimensional guided M-mode echocardiography. Can J Cardiol 2006; 23: 219–222.

[44] Harnett JD, Murphy B, Collingwood P, Purchase L, Kent G, Parfrey PS. The reliability and validity of echocardiographic measurement of left ventricular mass index in hemodialysis patients. Nephron 1993; 65: 3

[45] Martin LC, Barretti P, Cornejo IV, Felipe MJ, Forti AH, Matsubara BB, Okoshi K, Padovani CR, Teixeira-Caramori J, Ferreira Tucci PJ, da Silva Franco RJ. Influence of fluid volume variations on the calculated value of left ventricular mass measured by echocardiogram in patients submitted to hemodialysis. Ren Fail 2003; 25: 43–53

[46] Stewart GA, Foster J, Cowan M, Rooney E, McDonagh T, Dargie HJ, Rodger RS, Jardine AG. Echocardiography overestimates left ventricular mass in hemodialysis patients relative to magnetic resonance imaging. Kidney Int 1999; 56: 2248–2253.

In: Peritoneal Dialysis
Editors: A. Agarwal, L. Salman et al.
ISBN: 978-1-62257-896-2

Chapter 6

PERITONEAL DIALYSIS AND HYPERGLYCEMIA

*Ajay Yadlapati**, *Katherine Wu, Ephantus Njue, John Schomberg and Anjay Rastogi*
Division of Nephrology, Department of Medicine, UCLA,RR UCLA MC Los Angeles, California, US

ABSTRACT

Peritoneal Dialysis (PD) has seen rapid development and acceptance as a viable choice for acute and chronic dialysis over the last 25 years. Today, PD garners approx. 16% [1] of the chronic dialysis population and is expected to grow in the near future. This growth has allowed a larger patient demographic to utilize this service, one of those being diabetics. Conventional strategies have been diet and weight restrictions as well as using non glucose PD solutions such as icodextrin in combination with fewer daily exchanges of low-glucose solutions. Yet, no specific literature is present regarding the effects of various compositions of dialysate glucose solutions, nor a protocol to help distinguish when to use certain products.

* E-mail address: Ayadlapati@mednet.ucla.edu

Diabetic PD Patients and Risk of New-Onset Hyperglycemia

Currently, about 30% of all new dialysis patients are diabetics. Compared to non-diabetics on continuous ambulatory peritoneal dialysis (CAPD), both insulin-dependent and non-insulin-dependent diabetic patients are more vulnerable to comorbidities such as retinopathy, neuropathy and cardio-vascular diseases which ultimately lead to decreased survival. The Diabetes Control and Complications Trial (DCCT) found that hyperglycemia is the single main cause of this higher rate of complications [2]. Appropriate insulin regimens will therefore have the potential to reduce incidence and progression of complications.

The glycemic control of patients even before starting peritoneal dialysis has been found to reduce the rate of complications in type II diabetic ESRD patients on CAPD. Pre-dialysis glycemic control has been shown to be an independent prognostic predictor of clinical outcome in diabetics on CAPD [3]. Poor glycemic control is largely attributed to poor compliance, underlying comorbid conditions and possible insulin resistance.

Solutions used in peritoneal dialysis contain glucose concentrations ranging from 1360 to 3860mg/dl [4] and absorption of these solutions may play a part in potential hyperglycemia. Studies show that patients on peritoneal dialysis will absorb 70% of the glucose load through their abdominal cavity and gain 20% of their daily caloric energy from glucose in the dialysate. The aggregate amount of glucose rapidly absorbed from the peritoneal cavity can average the equivalent intake of 100 – 300g of glucose per day. Glucose absorption through the peritoneum has been found to result in significantly higher serum glucose levels than from an equivalent dose of oral dextrose [5]. This increased glucose load during PD has been associated with insulin resistance leading to hyperglycemia, dyslipidemia and hypertriglyceridemia [6].

Studies have found a large number of patients who develop new-onset hyperglycemia after initiation of PD [7]. Patients on PD have significantly higher glycated hemoglobin (Hb1A1C), fasting glucose and homeostasis model assessment (HOMA) index values compared with patients on hemodialysis [8]. Patients with non-diabetic nephropathy on extended continuous ambulatory peritoneal dialysis show dynamic fluctuations of fasting blood glucose, especially with continual or prolonged usage. A recent study showed that blood glucose levels were minimally changed at the end of the third month of CAPD, however, glucose levels were significantly elevated after both six and twelve months after initiation of PD [9]. Therefore, sustained use of a glucose medium in PD can predispose the patient to both hyperglycemia and the possible development of diabetes mellitus.

EFFECTS OF HYPERGLYCEMIA ON PD PATIENTS

D-Glucose has been used successfully for several decades as the osmotic agent employed in dialysis solutions to achieve adequate fluid removal. The absorption of 100-200 grams of glucose per day has been suggested as potentially increasing cardiometabolic risk, particularly in patients with diabetes [10]. Complications of hyperglycemia may accelerate with treatment using conventional glucose-containing solutions, including a (weak) 1.5% dextrose PD solution versus (strong) 4.25% dextrose PD solution. As stated before, recent studies showed that after PD initiation, a large number of patients developed new-onset hyperglycemia because of their exposure to hypertonic glucose solutions [11].

The disadvantages of glucose include its rapid dissipation from the peritoneum, the associated metabolic response to absorbed glucose in all patients, and the local effects of glucose, glucose degradation products, and hyperosmolality on peritoneal membrane structure and function. Similar to diabetes, glucose can contribute to peritoneal membrane failure possibly through the generation of glucose degradation products (GDPs) or the formation of advanced glycation end products (AGEs) [12. 13]. In addition, sterilization of conventional single-chamber glucose PD solutions at high temperature and relatively high pH (5.5) promotes generation of toxic GDP which impair peritoneal mesothelial cell function, affect local host defense mechanisms, and induce pro-angiogenic factors [14].

The effects of hyperglycemia on the body are vast and significant. Cardiovascular disease is the main cause of death in PD patients. This may partially be explained by preexisting risk factors such as anemia, uremia, dyslipidemia, malnutrition, vitamin D deficiency, excess parathyroid hormone and metabolic acidosis. However, the development of insulin resistance in PD patients after an initial improvement is generally attributed to the high levels of glucose absorbed from dialysate which contribute to metabolic abnormalities such as poor glycemic control, new-onset diabetes, central obesity, hypertension and hypertriglyceridemia [15]. Together, these metabolic derangements stimulate an inflammatory cascade, resulting in a rise in reactive oxygen species (ROS) production by mitochondria, which in turn activate serine-threonine kinases such as Jun N-terminal kinase (JNK) and inhibitor of NF-kB kinase. The overall effect of this cascade is the enhancement of insulin resistance and further development of metabolic abnormalities.

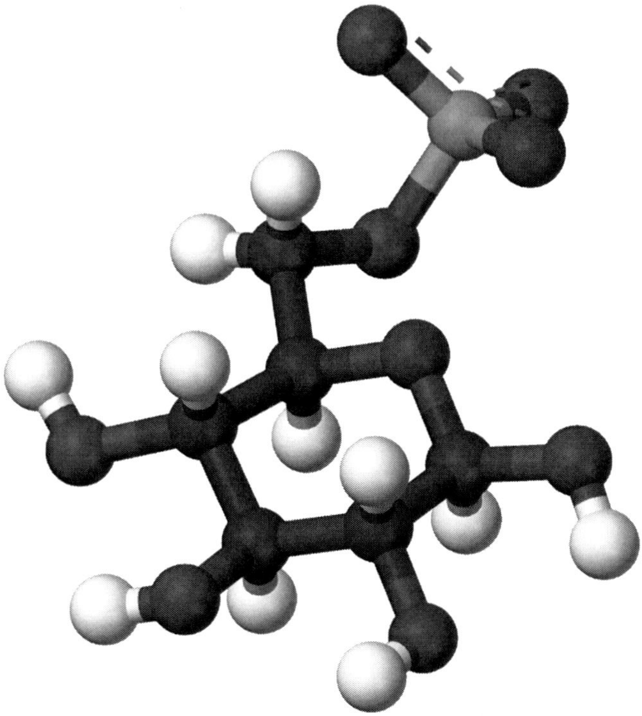

Figure 1. D-Glucose Molecular Structure.

The effect of glucose absorption appears to be amplified as a consequence of changes in the peritoneum and reduced ultrafiltration. A study examining the morphologic features of peritoneal membranes of 130 patients undergoing PD found vascular changes which were absent in normal subjects. These changes, resembling changes observed in diabetic microvascular disease, include reduplication of capillary basement membranes, expansion of extracellular matrix within the media of arterioles, deposition of type IV collagen within arterial walls and deposition of advanced glycosylation end products in vessel walls, resulting in luminal narrowing or obliteration [16]. In the PD group, the prevalence and severity of vasculopathy increased significantly with the duration of therapy. Additionally, the median thickness of the submesothelial compact collagenous zone was significantly increased when compared to hemodialysis patients as well as normal subjects. These vascular changes in peritoneal membranes of PD patients result in increased clearance of solute but also in more rapid glucose uptake.

In a large-scale study by Duong [17] 2,798 diabetic patients on dialysis were analyzed and found to have an association with higher all-class mortality and Hemoglobin A1C values greater than 8% as well as serum glucose greater than 300mg/dl. However, another study [18] failed to demonstrate this relationship between hemoglobin A1C and 1-year survival. Recent observational studies have shown the association of hemodialysis patients with lower cumulative survival in patient with poor glycemic control [19, 20]. More specifically, this relationship was also shown in the peritoneal dialysis subset [21]. The postulated mechanisms of this relationship may be related to microvascular complications, possibly due to the creation of advanced glycation end products (AGEs). Another factor that must be considered is the association of comorbidities and its predisposition to higher mortality rather than due to poor glycemic control solely [22]. In PD patients, higher A1C levels may contribute to damage to the peritoneal membrane secondary to the elevated cumulative glucose levels. This damage may be similar to microvascular disease found in diabetics, where the process of neovascularization may occur and ultimately lead to reduced ultrafiltration capacity.

The effects of hyperglycemia at the molecular level are vast. Many studies have demonstrated alterations in complement synthesis and inflammatory mediators such as monocyte chemo-attractant protein-1 (MCP-1) and transforming growth factor beta (TGF-b) [23]. Additionally, elevated glucose concentrations have been linked to the down-regulation of E-cadherin as well as a reduction of perlecan synthesis (an anionic heparan sulfate proteoglycan) that may alter the selective permeability of the peritoneal membrane [24, 25].

In equilibrium states, glucose is phosphorylated by hexokinase to glucose-6-phosphates. However in the setting of high glucose concentrations, glucose is converted to sorbitol by the enzyme aldose reductase. Certain literature has proposed that the intracellular accumulation of sorbitol and the subsequent conversion to fructose by sorbitol dehydrogenase, may be a potential cause of cellular dysfunction [26, 27]. The generation of fructose is coupled to NAD reduction, which has been postulated as enhancing the formation of diacylglycerol (DAG), which in turn stimulates protein kinase C (PKC) and contributes to diabetic tissue injury [28, 29].

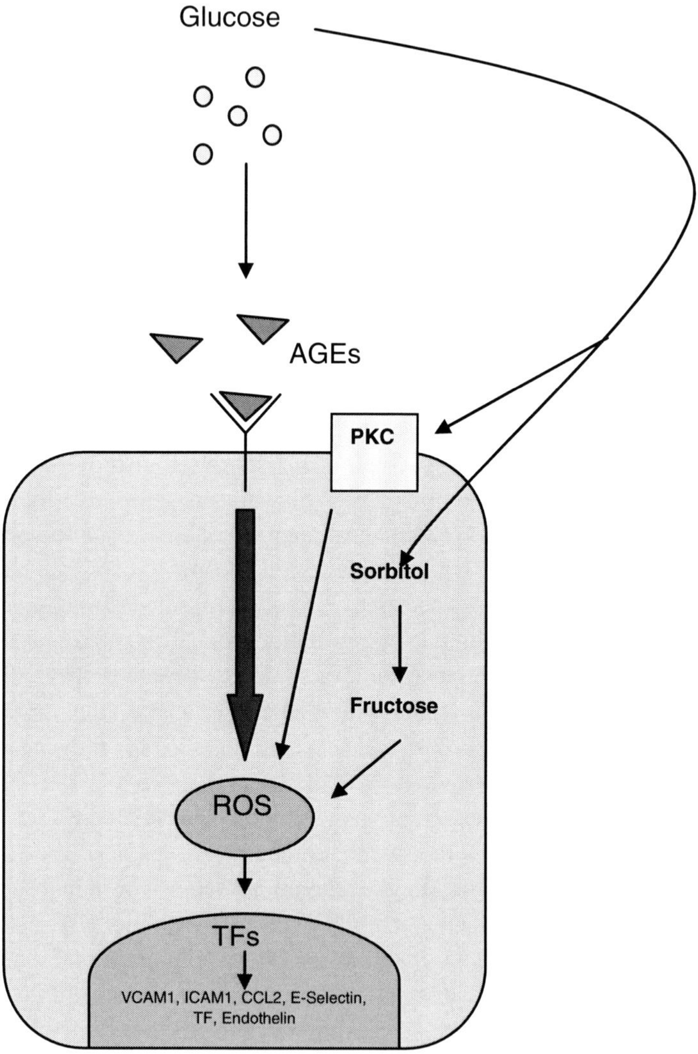

Figure 2. Intracellular Effects of Glucose – The creation of advanced glycation end-products (AGEs) by glucose can directly stimulates AGE receptors which lead to the development multiple signaling pathways. Glucose can also stimulate signaling pathways directly on Protein Kinase C (PKC) or through the sorbitol pathway. These pathways then generate reactive oxygen species (ROS) which ultimately affect transcription factors (TFs) at the molecular level.

Additionally, elevated glucose and hyperosmolar solutions have been shown to inhibit wound healing after peritoneal injury. Many other types of cells have also been shown to be affected by this environment including adipocytes, leukocytes, fibroblasts, and peritoneal vascular endothelial cells [30]. Recent evidence in rat models has shown structural and functional microvasculature alterations in the peritoneal membrane secondary to hyperglycemia. These changes include increased vascular density and elevated transport of small solutes with a concurrent increased expression of vascular endothelial growth factor (VEGF).

ICODEXTRIN

Icodextrin was recently introduced this last decade as a feasible alternative to conventional dextrose solutions for the once-daily long-dwell exchange in PD. It is effective, generally well tolerated and appears to be most useful in situations of reduced or inadequate ultrafiltration (UF) with dextrose, including in high and high-average transporters, during episodes of peritonitis and in patients who have failed dextrose-based dialysis. The tolerability of icodextrin was generally similar to that of dextrose-based solutions in controlled clinical trials, although there was an approximate three-fold increase in the risk of new skin rash [31].

Icodextrin is a high molecular weight glucose polymer developed specifically for use as an alternative osmotic agent to dextrose during the once-daily long-dwell exchange in peritoneal dialysis. Icodextrin induces transcapillary ultrafiltration by a mechanism similar to colloid osmosis. The GDP content and pH of icodextrin are low, while lactate concentration is high.

Although absorption of icodextrin from the peritoneal cavity is slower than conventional dextrose, 40-45% of icodextrin molecules are still absorbed in children and adults within 12-14 hours [32]. Once absorbed, icodextrin is metabolized to maltose and its derivatives which ultimately accumulate in the body and increase serum osmolality by 5 mosmol/L [33]. In children, the caloric load associated with a single daytime dwell of 600 mLm^2 of icodextrin is below 5% of the daily allowance of energy and after discontinuation of icodextrin, plasma levels of metabolites return to baseline within 3-7 days [34]. However, the long-term metabolic effects of icodextrin in a growing and developing child are unknown.

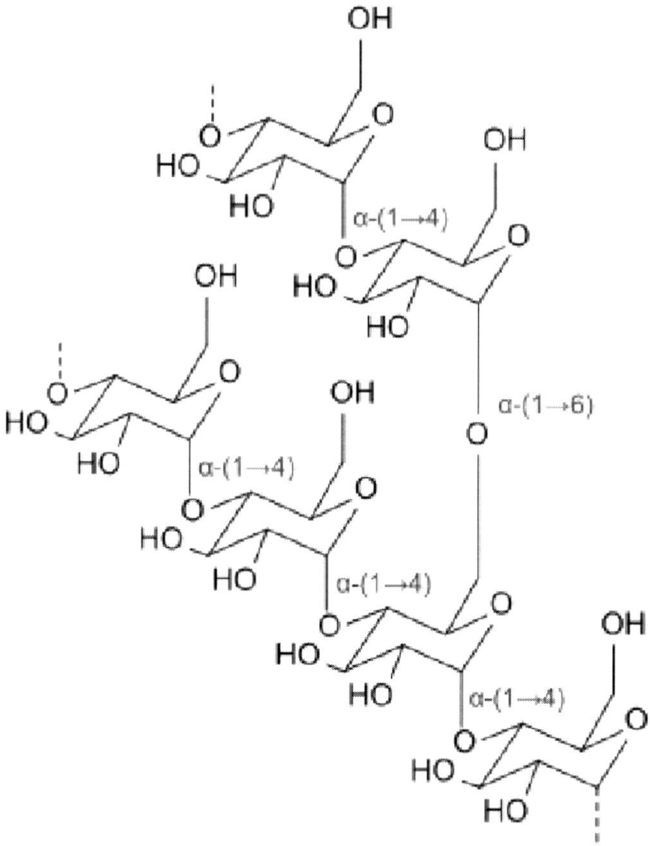

Figure 3. Icodextrin Molecular Structure

The slower absorption rate of icodextrin ultimately leads to longer ultrafiltration times as well as a lower carbohydrate load. The ultrafiltration pattern is delayed compared with standard dextrose PD fluids and the sustained net fluid withdrawal time of more than 12 hours largely prevents back-filtration [35]. Both local and systemic glucose load have been found to be significantly reduced with icodextrin usage and plasma lipid profile also has shown improvement [36]. Icodextrin administration during daytime dwell in adult patients has been shown to have better preserved peritoneal membrane function compared with that of conventional high-GDP solution [37]. Furthermore, studies have shown the long-term use of icodextrin to be associated with a decrease in the deterioration of membrane function [38, 39].

Two recent prospective, multicenter open-labeled studies by Paniagua [40] and Finkelstein [41] have reported that a significant HbA1C reduction could be achieved with icodextrin use. The most recent of these, by Paniagua, was a randomized controlled study of 59 diabetic CAPD patients with a 12-month follow-up period, where HbA1C values rose by 0.79% in the glucose-only group versus a fall of 0.98% in the icodextrin group, which was clinically significant [42].

Some disadvantages of icodextrin solution result from the high lactate concentration and low pH. Icodextrin can only be used once daily as its lactate based buffered PD solution can cause a buildup of lactate. In addition, allergic skin reactions following icodextrin administration have been reported in up to 10% of patients.

Alternative Strategies to Reduce Hyperglycemia

The double-chamber system employs the principle of two separate bags; one containing a concentrated glucose solution kept at a low pH and a larger compartment containing the electrolyte/buffer solution. Just prior to use, the two compartments are mixed to create normal therapeutic concentrations of glucose and a physiologic pH. The double-chamber design is based upon the idea that high glucose concentrations at an acidic pH result in lower GDP generation and ultimately a decreased amount of AGEs produced in the peritoneal cavity [43]. The lower GDP concentration may help to better preserve the functional integrity of the peritoneal membrane [44]. Numerous research and clinical studies have demonstrated that multi-chamber PD fluids indeed have improved biocompatibility profiles compared with single-chamber fluids [45].

In vitro, multi-chamber PD fluids preserve innate peritoneal immune defense mechanisms, improve mesothelial cell viability and function and reduce synthesis and secretion of inflammatory and angiogenic cytokines. Animal studies also confirm improved preservation of the mesothelial cell layer, reduced peritoneal TGF-B and VEGF expression, reduced deposition of AGE and reduced fibrosis, vasculopathy and negoangiogenesis [46]. In humans, long term trials in PD patients found better preservation of renal function with the use of multi-chamber fluids possibly due to reduced resorption of toxic GDP [47]. Clinical benefits of multi-chamber PD fluids also include reduced abdominal discomfort due to the reduction of intraperitoneal pressure and inflow pain [48]. Overall, single chamber bags have fallen out of favor due to augmented proliferation of GDPs and AGEs, which as a consequence can hinder the functional integrity of the peritoneal membrane.

Another mechanism of reducing GDP formation in PD solution is via sterilization by filtration. This is thought to aid in cell viability [49]. The sterilization process generates a large number of glucose degradation products. The filtering procedure avoids the undesirable glucose degradation as long as the fluids are not stored for long periods of time [50].

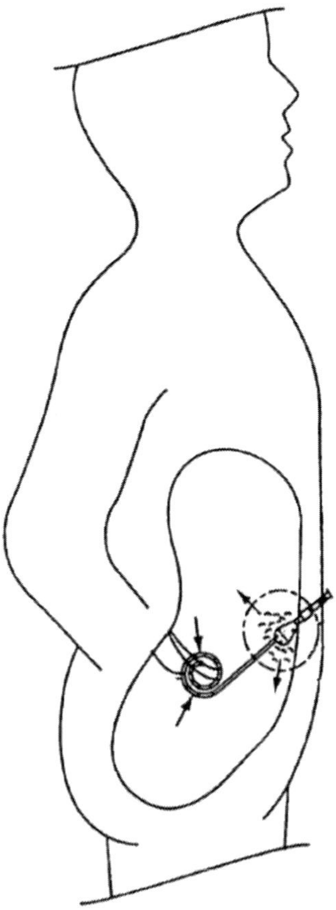

Figure 4. Continuous Flow PD - A modality in which continuous circulation of PD fluid is maintained at a high flow rate using two separate catheters or one dual-lumen catheter.

Additionally, continuous-flow PD is another potential way to reduce glucose load. This modality works via the mechanism of large constant intraperitoneal volumes of fluids which are either replenished through a single circuit, through recirculation of dialysate through an external regenerating apparatus, or by maximizing the transperitoneal solute gradient. In essence, this process allows an effective osmotic gradient to be maintained with a very low glucose gradient.

As mentioned above, the replacement of glucose with other osmolar agents has also been utilized. This method has shown benefit in preservation of ultrastructure, viability, and protein synthesis compared with conventional glucose-based PD fluids [51]. The use of these alternatives must be weighed against the risk of excessive nitrogen load, thus cannot be applied to replace all PD exchanges. Additionally, these solutions may impair endothelial function, which may increase the risk of cardiovascular disease. These compounds have also been shown to reduce activation of the peritoneal immune system, peritoneal neo-angiogenesis, fibrosis, and damage to mesothelial cells which aid in the formation of a protective barrier against invading particulates (MCs) [52].

Table 1. Types of PD Solutions

	Dextrose	Amino Acid	Icodextrin
Molecular Weight (Daltons)	182	100-200	20,000
Osmolality (mOsm/kg)	346-485	365	282
Complications	Hyper insulinemia, hyperglycemia, hyperlipidemia, and weight gain	Cost, Acidosis, Increase nitrogen burden	Rise in maltose, maltotriose, and oligopolysacharides

Current Standard of Care for Hyperglycemic Patients on Dialysis

Hemoglobin A1C has become the standard in measuring glycemic control in the patient population. Poor glycemic control, indicated by high HbA1C levels, is associated with adverse outcomes, including prolonged hospitalization and shortened survival, in diabetics on PD [53]. HbA1C is the largest fraction formed and the most consistent index of the prevailing ambient concentration of circulating glucose.

Newly created hemoglobin in red blood cells has very little glucose attachment initially; however glucose becomes irreversibly attached based upon the circulating glucose concentration. Therefore, the hemoglobin A1C illustrates the mean blood glucose concentration over the erythrocyte lifespan of approximately 120 days. Glycation of hemoglobin occurs throughout the 120-day average lifetime of red blood cells with the oldest cells being the most glycated, and the youngest, the least glycated [54].

With more rapid red cell turnover in hemodialysis patients, a greater proportion of younger red cells will be present in the circulation. This is of particular importance in patients on HD therapy, in whom RBC life span is shortened by approximately 50% [55, 56]. These younger cells will have a lower initial glucose attachment, thereby leading to falsely low A1C values.

Although dialysis may lend to a falsely low HbA1C, other factors can alter this value as well. Elevated blood urea nitrogen leads to the formation of carbamylated hemoglobin. Elevated urea levels in patients with renal failure may dissociate in the circulation to form cyanate, which in its reactive form condenses with the N-terminal amino groups of hemoglobin in a process similar to glycation to form carbamylated hemoglobin [57, 58]. Carbamylated hemoglobin forms by dissociation of urea to cyanate and condensation of cyanate with hemoglobin. This molecule is then read as glyosylated hemoglobin by certain electrical charge based assays. This artificial elevation in HbA1C must be considered in all renal patients as well [59].

Table 2. HbA1C Effects

Factors Affecting HbA1C	
Decrease	**Increase**
Iron Deficiency Anemia	Elevated BUN
Recent Transfusion	
Epo Stimulating Agents	
Hemodialysis	

Many other factors also contribute to alterations in HbA1C values such as iron deficiency, recent transfusion, and use of erythropoietin stimulating agents which all may also cause underestimation of glucose control [60]. Overall the main impact of dialysis on HbA1C is a falsely low or underestimation; which may impact diabetic management.

Current Practice in the Management of Hyperglycemia Patients through Dietary Interventions

Managing diabetic patients' hyperglycemia through dietary intervention is not a practice of care unique to the modality of peritoneal dialysis. It is important that the registered dietitian managing the care of these patients be aware of the greater risk of weight gain in non-diabetic patients on diabetes and the increased risk of diabetes for those patients with greater weight gain. Patients with a BMI >26 should be counseled on controlling caloric consumption to prevent further weight gain that would further decrease insulin sensitivity and increase risk of progression of diabetes.

Patients should be counseled and educated on assessing the content of carbohydrates in foods and dosing short acting insulin to act upon the carbohydrate consumed with each meal. Traditional carbohydrate restrictions for diabetic patients are 45-60g of carbohydrate/meal for women and 60-75g of carbohydrate/meal for men. Snacks in between meals should amount to no more than 15-30g of carbohydrate/snack. Patients should be counseled to avoid foods with high fat content and encouraged to include higher fiber foods. High fat foods tend to cause blood sugar spikes to stay at higher levels longer while high fiber foods tend to slow upward rise of blood sugar in diabetic patients while maintaining those lower peaks for longer periods of time when compared with patients on low fiber diets with equal carbohydrate content. Combining a diabetic diet with a renal diet is challenging but achievable. Training in the assessment of carbohydrate in foods in addition to assessing mineral content are important skills that will help the patient manage hyperglycemia and other components of long term care. There are many resources available to patients today providing patients with information on carbohydrate and mineral content of foods. As with all dietary interventions patients should have counseling tailored on an individual level allowing them to maintain as much of their personal and cultural practices as possible.

Assessing Patient Competence and Compliance

Behavior change and assessment is crucial in the management of care of patients with chronic disease. The medication and dietary regimens that healthcare practitioners prescribe to patients will only be effective if those patients choose to adopt the changes recommended by doctors, nurses, and dietitians. The team should work together in using standardized tests to assess the patient's ability to perform complex tasks related to their care. In some cases if the patient is cared for by a friend or family member the caretaker should also be assessed for competence and care should be planned to accommodate individual competence levels of the patient or caretaker. Domains tested should be reported interest, motivation, ability to verbalize instructions, family support, and reported compliance. Competence should be reevaluated bi-annually so that care may be refocused to best meet patient needs. Incorporating technology into patient care such as an insulin pump and glucose sensor technology are methods of treatment whose adoption should be strongly influenced by the level of patient or caretaker competence.

Insulin Administration

Appropriate insulin treatment to improve glycemic control in hyperglycemic PD patients has the potential to reduce incidence and progression of complications. During peritoneal dialysis, glycemic control is made more difficult by the additional supply of glucose via the peritoneum. Furthermore, patients on intermittent peritoneal dialysis (IPD) have the added problem of the discontinuous quality of additional glucose supply. The goal of insulin treatment during PD is to maintain euglycemia during the dwell time, preventing postprandial hyperglycemia and morning hypoglycemia. Various forms of insulin administration include intraperitoneal administration, subcutaneous administration and oral administration of hypoglycemic agents. A recent study has shown that CAPD patients are mostly treated with insulin, while less than 4% with oral hypoglycemic agents. More specifically, more than half of CAPD patients receive their insulin via an intraperitoneal route [61].

Intraperitoneal administration of insulin has been found to result in more rapid and even absorption compared with subcutaneous administration. In PD, with the addition of insulin to dialysis fluid, insulin is absorbed continuously throughout the entire dwell time. Insulin administered via the intraperitoneal route passes directly into the portal vein system and influences glucose and lipid metabolism from the liver, selectively inhibiting excessively high hepatic glucose release. In patients without diabetes, the liver will metabolize 50-70% of the insulin absorbed through the peritoneal membrane. The degree of hyperinsulinemia is less than with subcutaneous administration, as the amount of insulin reaching the periphery is much less. This is important because the level of circulating insulin has been directly correlated with the risk of arteriosclerosis [62].

The adsorption of insulin to the polyvinyl chloride surfaces of dialysis fluid bags and tubing is another factor to be taken into consideration. It has been found that approximately 10% of added insulin bound to the polyvinyl chloride reservoirs after the first minute of administration and approximately 20% bound after 15 minutes. The amount of insulin adsorbed correlated directly with the total surface area of the reservoir and inversely with the insulin concentration of the dialysis fluid [63].

In CAPD, the intraperitoneal insulin requirement was less if insulin was administered into empty abdominal cavity before the instillation of dialysis fluid. A higher insulin dose was required when insulin was infused with the dialysis fluid into the abdominal cavity. The blood glucose values also fluctuated less with intraperitoneal than with subcutaneous administration. However when dialysis fluids with glucose concentrations higher than 13.6 g/L are used, the absorption of glucose is greater in both CAPD and IPD with intraperitoneal insulin treatment than with subcutaneous administration. When the absorption of insulin from dialysis solution instilled in three CAPD patients with diabetes was compared with the absorption in three CAPD without, absorption of insulin in patients with diabetes was much higher than in patients without diabetes after a dwell time of 30 minutes [64].

A recent study illustrated that the instillation of insulin into the abdominal cavity before introduction of dialysis fluid had lower amounts of total insulin use and lower HbA1C levels. These results were consistent with an earlier study in which a fall of HbA1C from an average of 10.6 to 8.3% was observed after switching from subcutaneous to intraperitoneal insulin administration [65].

Subcutaneous insulin administration results in major fluctuations in blood glucose values due to different rates of insulin degradation after leaving subcutaneous tissues dependent on the position and depth of injection, regional blood flow and physical exertion [66]. Therefore, the utilization of insulin through the intraperitoneum route may be advantageous in the glycemic control of peritoneal patients.

Peritoneal dialysis will continue to grow in the near future as a viable choice for acute and chronic dialysis. Concurrent with its growth is the expansion of the patient demographic, including more glucose intolerance or diabetic patients. Therefore, more consideration must be given to the composition of PD solutions regarding their glycemic effects. Numerous modalities are available to help curtail hyperglycemia in these patients, including the use of icodextrin, dual-chamber system, solution sterilization, continuous-flow PD, insulin administration and more. Appropriate management of these PD solutions will ultimately have the potential to reduce incidence and progression of diabetic complications.

REFERENCES

[1] Ganter G: On the elimination of toxic substances from the blood by dialysis. Munch Med Wochenschr 1923; 70: 1478-1488.

[2] The Diabetes Control and Complications Trial Research Group. The Effect of Intensive Treatment of Diabetes on the Development and Progression of Long-Term Complications in Insulin-Dependent Diabetes Mellitus. N Engl J Med 1993; 329:977-986September 30, 1993.

[3] Yu CC, Wu MS, Wu CH, Yang CW, Huang JY, Hong JJ, Fan Chiang CY, Leu ML, Huang CC. Predialysis glycemic control is an independent predictor of clinical outcome in type II diabetics on continuous ambulatory peritoneal dialysis. Perit Dial Int. 1997 May-Jun;17(3):262-8.

[4] Duong U. Glycemic control and survical in peritoneal dialysis patients with diabetes mellitus. Clin J Am Soc Nephrol. 6: 1041-1048, 2011.

[5] FortesPC, Mendes JG, Riella MC, Pecoits–Filho R. Carbohydrate metabolism disturbances in non-diabetic patients on peritoneal dialysis. Perit Dial Int 2006; 26 (Suppl 2):S26.

[6] Gallieni M, Musetti C, Granata A, Olivi L, Bertoli S. Metabolic consequences of peritoneal dialysis treatment.Panminerva Med. 2009 Sep;51(3):175-85. Review

[7] Szeto CC, Chow KM, Kwan BC, Chung KY, Leung CB, Li PK. New-onset hyperglycemia in nondiabetic Chinese patients started on peritoneal dialysis. Am J Kidney Dis 2007; 49: 524–32.

[8] Fortes PC, de Moraes TP, Mendes JG, Stinghen AE, Ribeiro SC, Pecoits-Filho R. Insulin resistance and glucose homeostasis in peritoneal dialysis.Perit Dial Int. 2009 Feb;29 Suppl 2:S145-8. Review.

[9] Yu XF, Zhou YF, Feng L, Zhang DL, Liu WH. Influence of peritoneal transfer status on fasting blood glucose in non-diabetic nephropathy patients on continuous ambulatory peritoneal dialysis. Chin Med J (Engl). 2009 Dec 20;122(24):2977-80.

[10] Holmes CJ. Reducing cardiometabolic risk in peritoneal dialysis patients: role of the dialysis solution. J Diabetes Sci Technol. 2009 Nov 1;3(6):1472-80.

[11] Szeto CC, Chow KM, Kwan BC, Chung KY, Leung CB, Li PK. New-onset hyperglycemia in nondiabetic Chinese patients started on peritoneal dialysis. Am J Kidney Dis 2007; 49:524–32.

[12] Ha H, Lee HB. Effect of high glucose on peritoneal mesothelial cell biology. Perit Dial Int 2000; 20(Suppl 2): S15–18.

[13] Sitter T, Sauter M. Impact of glucose in peritoneal dialysis: saint or sinner? Peritoneal Dialysis International, Vol. 25, pp. 415–425

[14] Schmitt CP, Bakkaloglu SA, Klaus G, Schröder C, Fischbach M. Solutions for peritoneal dialysis in children: recommendations by the European Pediatric Dialysis Working Group. Pediatr Nephrol. 2011 Jul;26(7):1137-47. Epub 2011 Mar 31.

[15] FortesPC,MendesJG,RiellaMC,Pecoits–FilhoR. Carbohydrate metabolism disturbances in non-diabetic patients on peritoneal dialysis. Perit Dial Int 2006; 26 (Suppl 2):S26.

[16] Williams JD, Craig KJ, Topley N, Von Ruhland C, Fallon M, Newman GR, Mackenzie RK, Williams GT (2002) Morphologic changes in the peritoneal membrane of patients with renal disease. J Am Soc Nephrol 13:470–479

[17] Duong U. Glycemic control and survical in peritoneal dialysis patients with diabetes mellitus. Clin J Am Soc Nephrol. 6: 1041-1048, 2011.

[18] Williams ME, Larson E Jr., Teng M, Ofsthun N, Lazarus JM: Hemodialzyed type I and type II diabetic patients in the US; Characteristics, glycemic control, and survival. Kidney Int 70: 1503-1509, 2006.

[19] Wu MS, Yu CC, Yang CW, Wu CH, Huang JY, Hong JJ, Fan Chiang CY, Huang CC, Leu ML: Poor pre-dialysis glycemic control is a predictor of mortality in type II diabetic patients on maintanence hemodialsyis. Nephrol Dial Transplant 12: 2105-2110, 1997.

[20] Kalantar-Zadeh K, Kopple JD, Regidor DL, Jing J, Shinaberger CS, Aronovitz J, McAllister CJ, Whellan D, Sharma K: A1C and survival in maintanence hemodialysis patients. Diabetes Care 30: 1049-1055, 2007.
[21] Wu MS, Yu CC, Wu CH, Haung JY, Leu ML, Huang CC: Pre-dialysis glycemic control is an independant predictor of mortality in type II diabetic patients on continous ambuatory peritoneal dialsyis. Perit Dial Int 19 [Suppl 2]: S179-S183, 1999.
[22] Duong U. Glycemic control and survical in peritoneal dialysis patients with diabetes mellitus. Clin J Am Soc Nephrol. 6: 1041-1048, 2011.
[23] Wong TY, Phillips AO, Witowski J, Topley N. Glucose-mediated induction of TGF-beta 1 and MCP-1 in mesothelial cells in vitro is osmolality and polyol pathway dependent. Kidney Int 2003; 63:1404–16.
[24] Yanez-Mo M, Lara-Pezzi E, Selgas R, Ramirez-Huesca M, Dominguez-Jimenez C, Jimenez-Hefferman JA, et al. Peritoneal dialysis and epithelial-to-mesenchymal transition of mesothelial cells. N Engl J Med 2003; 348:403–13.
[25] Yung S, Chen XR, Tsang RC, Zhang Q, Chan TM. Reduction of perlecan synthesis and induction of TGF-beta1 in human peritoneal mesothelial cells due to high dialysate glucose concentration: implication in peritoneal dialysis. J Am Soc Nephrol 2004; 15:1178–88.
[26] Morrisey K, Steadman R, Williams JD, Phillips AO. Renal proximal tubular cell fibronectin accumulation in response to glucose is polyol pathway dependent. Kidney Int 1999; 55:160–7.
[27] Brownlee M. Biochemistry and molecular cell biology of diabetic complications. Nature 2001; 414:813–20.
[28] Tilton RG, Baier LD, Harlow JE, Smith SR, Ostrow E, Williamson JR. Diabetes-induced glomerular dysfunction: links to a more reduced cytosolic ratio of NADH/NAD+. Kidney Int 1992; 41:778–88.
[29] Craven PA, Davidson CM, DeRubertis FR. Increase in diacylglycerol mass in isolated glomeruli by glucose from de novo synthesis of glycerolipids. Diabetes 1990; 39:667–74.
[30] Tamura M, Osajima A, Nakayamada S, Anai H, Kabashima N, Kanegae K, et al. High glucose levels inhibit focal adhesion kinase-mediated wound healing of rat peritoneal mesothelial cells. Kidney Int 2003; 63:722–31
[31] Frampton JE, Plosker GL. Icodextrin: a review of its use in peritoneal dialysis. Drugs. 2003;63(19):2079-105.

[32] Moberly JB, Mujais S, Gehr T, Hamburger R, Sprague S, Kucharski A, Reynolds R, Ogrinc F, Martis L, Wolfson M (2002) Pharmacokinetics of icodextrin in peritoneal dialysis patients. Kidney Int Suppl 81:S23–S33

[33] Posthuma N, ter Wee PM, Donker AJ, Oe PL, Peers EM, Verbrugh HA, The Dextrin in APD in Amsterdam (DIANA) Group (2000) Assessment of the effectiveness, safety, and biocompatibility of icodextrin in automated peritoneal dialysis. Perit Dial Int 20 [Suppl 2]:S106–S113

[34] Canepa A, Verrina E, Perfumo F (2008) Use of new peritoneal dialysis solutions in children. Kidney Int Suppl 108:S137–S144

[35] Michallat AC, Dheu C, Loichot C, Danner S, Fischbach M (2005) Long daytime exchange in children on continuous cycling peritoneal dialysis: preservation of drained volume because of icodextrin use. Adv Perit Dial 21:195–199

[36] Bredie SJ, Bosch FH, Demacker PN, Stalenhoef AF, van Leusen R (2001) Effects of peritoneal dialysis with an overnight icodextrin dwell on parameters of glucose and lipid metabolism. Perit Dial Int 21:275–281

[37] Davies SJ, Brown EA, Frandsen NE, Rodrigues AS, Rodriguez-Carmona A, Vychytil A, Macnamara E, Ekstrand A, Tranaeus A, Filho JC, EAPOS Group (2005) Longitudinal membrane function in functionally anuric patients treated with APD: data from EAPOS on the effects of glucose and icodextrin prescrip- tion. Kidney Int 67:1609–1615

[38] Frampton J., Plosker G. Icodextrin: A Review of its Use in Peritoneal Dialysis. Drugs 2003; 63 (19): 2079-2105

[39] Davies SJ, Brown EA, Frandsen NE, Rodrigues AS, Rodriguez-Carmona A, Vychytil A, et al. Longitudinal membrane function in functionally anuric patients treated with APD: data from EAPOS on the effects of glucose and icodextrin prescription. Kidney Int 2005; 67:1609–15.

[40] Paniagua R, Ventura MD, Avila-Diaz M, Cisneros A,Vicente-Martinez M, Furlong MD, Garcia-Gonzalez Z, Villanueva D, Orihuela O, Prado-Uribe MD, Alcantara G, Amato D. Icodextrin improves metabolic and fluid management in high and high-average transport diabetic patients. Perit Dial Int. 2009;29(4):422-32.

[41] Finkelstein F, Healy H, Abu-Alfa A, Ahmad S, Brown F, Gehr T, Nash K, Sorkin M, Mujais S.Superiority of icodextrin compared with 4.25% dextrose for peritoneal ultrafiltration.J Am Soc Nephrol. 2005 Feb;16(2):546-54. Epub 2004 Dec 29.

[42] Paniagua R, Ventura MD, Avila-Diaz M, Cisneros A,Vicente-Martinez M, Furlong MD, Garcia-Gonzalez Z, Villanueva D, Orihuela O, Prado-Uribe MD, Alcantara G, Amato D. Icodextrin improves metabolic and fluid management in high and high-average transport diabetic patients. Perit Dial Int. 2009;29(4):422-32.

[43] Ledebo I, Wieslander A, Kjellstrand P. Can we prevent the degradation of glucose in peritoneal dialysis solutions? Perit Dial Int 2000; 20(Suppl 2):S48–51.

[44] Jutta Passlick–Deetjen, Et. Al. In Vitro Superiority of Dual-Chambered Peritoneal Dialysis Solution with Possible Clinical Benefits. Peritoneal Dialysis International, Vol. 21 (2001), Supplement 3

[45] Schmitt CP, Bakkaloglu SA, Klaus G, Schröder C, Fischbach M. Solutions for peritoneal dialysis in children: recommendations by the European Pediatric Dialysis Working Group. Pediatr Nephrol. 2011 Jul;26(7):1137-47. Epub 2011 Mar 31.

[46] Mortier S, Faict D, Lameire NH, De Vriese AS (2005) Benefits of switching from a conventional to a low-GDP bicarbonate/ lactate-buffered dialysis solution in a rat model. Kidney Int 67:1559–1665

[47] Kim SG, Kim S, Hwang YH, Kim K, Oh JE, Chung W, Oh KH, Kim HJ, Ahn C, Group Korean Balnet Study (2008) Could solutions low in glucose degradation products preserve residual renal function in incident peritoneal dialysis patients. Perit Dial Int 28 [Suppl 3]:S117–S122

[48] Mactier RA, Sprosen TS, Gokal R, Williams PF, Lindbergh M, Naik RB, Wrege U, Gröntoft KC, Larsson R, Berglund J, Tranaeus AP, Faict D (1998) Bicarbonate and bicarbonate/lactate peritoneal dialysis solutions for the treatment of infusion pain. Kidney Int 53:1061–1067.

[49] Witowski J, Bender TO, Gahl GM, Frei U, Jorres A. Glucose degradation products and peritoneal membrane function. Perit Dial Int 2001; 21:201–5.

[50] Wieslander, AP., Kjellstrand P., Rippel B. Heat sterilization of glucose-containing fluids for peritoneal dialysis: Biological consequences of chemical alterations. Peritoneal Dialysis Int. Vol 15. No 7 Supp. 1995

[51] Chan TM, Leung JK, Sun Y, Lai KN, Tsang RC, Yung S. Different effects of amino acid-based and glucose-based dialysate from peritoneal dialysis patients on mesothelial cell ultrastructure and function. Nephrol Dial Transplant 2003; 18:1086–94.

[52] Zareie M, van Lambalgen AA, ter Wee PM, Hekking LH, Keuning ED, Schadee-Eestermans IL, et al. Better preservation of the peritoneum in

rats exposed to amino acidbased peritoneal dialysis fluid. Perit Dial Int 2005; 25: 58–67.

[53] Tzamaloukas AH. Interpreting glycosylated hemoglobin in diabetic patients on peritoneal dialysis. Adv Perit Dial. 1996;12:171-5.

[54] Fitzgibbons JF, Koler RD, Jones RT: Red cell agerelated changes in haemoglobin A1a 1b and A1C in normal individuals and diabetic subjects. J Clin Invest 58:820-824, 1976

[55] Ansari A, Thomas S, Goldsmith D. Assessing glycemic control in patients with diabetes and end-stage renal failure. American Journal of Kidney Diseases. Volume 41, Issue 3, March 2003, Pages 523-531

[56] Eschbach JW Jr, Funk D, Adamson J, Kuhn I, Scribner BH, Finch CA: Erythropoiesis in patients with renal failure undergoing chronic dialysis. N Engl J Med 276:653- 658, 1967

[57] Davenport A, Jones S, Goel S, Astley JP, Feest TG: Carbamylated hemoglobin: A potential marker for the adequacy of hemodialysis therapy in end-stage renal failure. Kidney Int 50:1344-1351, 1996

[58] Fluckiger R, HarmonW, MeierW, Loo S, Gabbay H: Hemoglobin carbamylation in uremia. N Engl J Med 304: 823-827, 1981

[59] Tzamaloukas AH. Interpreting glycosylated hemoglobin in diabetic patients on peritoneal dialysis. Adv Perit Dial. 1996;12:171-5.

[60] Joy MS, Cefali WT, Hogan Sl, Nachman PH. Long-term glycemic control measurements in diabetic patients receiving hemodialysis. Am J Kidney Dis 2002; 39:297–307.

[61] Lindblad AS, Novak JW, Nolph KD, Stablein DM, Cutler SJ, Steinberg SM: Continuous Ambulatory Peritoneal Dialysis in the USA. Dordrecht, Kluwer, 1989, pp 63–74

[62] Quellhorst E. Insulin therapy during peritoneal dialysis: Pros and cons of various forms of administration. J Am Soc Nephrol. 2002 Jan;13 Suppl 1:S92-6.

[63] Johnson CA, Amidon G, Reichert JE, Porter WR: Adsorption of insulin to the surface of peritoneal dialysis solution containers. Am J Kidney Dis 3: 224–228, 1983

[64] Wideröe T, Smeby L et al. Long-Term Changes in Transperitoneal Water Transport during Continuous Ambulatory Peritoneal Dialysis. Nephron 1984;38:238-247

[65] Stephen RL, Maxwell JG, Harrow JJ, Jacobson SC, Hanover BK: Intervention in nephropathy due to insulin-dependent diabetes mellitus (IDDM). Kidney Int 28[Suppl 17]: S60–S65, 1985

[66] Quellhorst E. Insulin therapy during peritoneal dialysis: Pros and cons of various forms of administration. J Am Soc Nephrol. 2002 Jan;13 Suppl 1:S92-6.

INDEX

C

E

F

G

H

I

Q

R

S

W

X